No More Glasses

No More Glasses

◆

The Complete Guide to Laser Vision Correction

Julius Shulman, MD

Illustrations by Neil O. Hardy, FAMI

Graphic design—Barbara Zionce

iUniverse, Inc.

New York Lincoln Shanghai

No More Glasses
The Complete Guide to Laser Vision Correction

iUniverse books may be ordered through booksellers or by contacting:

iUniverse
2021 Pine Lake Road, Suite 100
Lincoln, NE 68512
www.iuniverse.com
1-800-Authors (1-800-288-4677)

ISBN-13: 978-0-595-35421-4 (pbk)
ISBN-13: 978-0-595-79916-9 (ebk)
ISBN-10: 0-595-35421-1 (pbk)
ISBN-10: 0-595-79916-7 (ebk)

Printed in the United States of America

To my family—at home and at work.

Contents

Acknowledgments

I wish to express my thanks to Tim Herrick, who helped jump-start this manuscript and undoubtedly learned more than he ever wished to know about laser vision correction. My friend, Jethro Lieberman, bespoke yet again, helped me immeasurably by giving up many nights and weekends to save me from the ignominy of my own writing. And special thanks go to my patients, whose quest for better vision inspired this revised edition.

Introduction

If you are reading this book, you probably wear glasses or contact lenses or know someone who does. You've probably heard about another option for vision correction—laser vision correction surgery (LVC). This option can mean an end to:

- Scrambling for your glasses to read the alarm clock or even to get out of bed.

- Searching for the soap in the shower because you can't see it.

- Being unable to see yourself in the mirror at the hair salon or barbershop.

- Eye irritation from keeping your contacts in too long because you don't have your glasses with you, and you can't take your contacts out until you get home.

- Passing up water sports and other activities because your corrective lenses make them impractical.

Millions of people have successfully undergone laser vision correction surgery. By reducing or eliminating their dependence on glasses and contact lenses, LVC has improved their quality of life. But is LVC the right choice for you? What do you need to know about your vision condition to make an informed decision about the procedure? If you are over forty, will you still need reading glasses? Will your astigmatism be corrected? How do you find the right doctor for the operation?

I've been an ophthalmologist since 1975, and eye health and vision correction have been my life's work. In the first edition of *No More Glasses* in 1987, I explored the most current vision correction surgical procedure—radial keratotomy (RK). Although it promised life without glasses, RK was limited to mild refractive errors and was somewhat unpredictable. In 1995, after years of scientific study and clinical trials and clinical trials conducted worldwide, the Food and Drug Administration approved the excimer laser—a new device for correcting vision, instantly making the riskier RK surgery almost obsolete. The excimer laser made possible three remarkable procedures—LASIK, PRK, and LASEK. These procedures are vastly safer and superior to RK, and to any other previous vision correction surgery. Results are more predictable, there are fewer complications, more types of vision errors can be corrected, and the healing time is shorter.

But with the evolution of laser vision correction (LVC) has come confusion. The marketing of LVC in various media has often minimized the medical nature of the procedure, emphasizing instead, the often miraculous improvement in vision. These mixed messages have often caused the non-discerning patient to equate LASIK, now almost a household word, with nonmedical purchases, such as buying a new shirt or a trip to the Bahamas, instead of the serious surgery that it really is.

This book will provide much of the information you will need to know about LVC and will help you decide if you are a good candidate for this operation. It will show how you can wake up each morning and see the clock on your nightstand, the trees outside your window, and the smiling face in the mirror—all without glasses or contacts.

In LVC, science, medicine, technology, and a physician's skill all converge to produce what is often a life-changing event—clarity of vision without glasses or contact lenses. LVC is an outpatient procedure that takes a few short minutes to perform and heals rapidly. But it is not simple and should not be taken lightly. It may be the most important decision you ever make. Such a decision must be intelligent and informed, requiring an understanding of how the eye works, the principles upon which the surgery is based, and the risks and complications every patient faces. Unlike the devices that compensate for myopia, hyperopia, or astigmatism, LVC can cure those vision conditions permanently.

The purpose of this book is patient education. Through a clear and simple appraisal of LVC, I hope to present the most current data in an understandable way and to enable you or someone you care about to make an informed decision about our most precious gift—the gift of sight. LVC may be within your reach, but you must know what awaits you and how to safely reach your goal of "no more glasses."

1

Laser Vision Correction Surgery—An Overview

During laser vision correction surgery, a computer-controlled laser removes (ablates) a thin layer of tissue from the cornea—the outer clear dome at the front of your eye. The ablation is done in a precise pattern, either flattening or steepening the cornea. By predictably changing the cornea's shape, your eye surgeon can cure such conditions as farsightedness, nearsightedness, and astigmatism and can eliminate or greatly reduce your need for glasses or contact lenses.

Three types of LVC are available: PRK (photorefractive keratectomy), approved in the United States for vision correction in 1995; LASIK (laser-assisted in situ keratomileusis), the most popular form of LVC, approved a few years later; and LASEK (laser sub-epithelial keratomileusis), a hybrid technique developed in 2002.

LVC has many acronyms, starting with the word laser—an acronym for light amplification by stimulated emission of radiation. Lasers, such as the argon laser to treat glaucoma and the ocular complications of diabetes on the eye, and the yag laser for post-cataract membranes, have been used in ophthalmology for over thirty years. The excimer laser—for vision correction surgery—is more recent. It was developed by IBM in the 1970s to etch microcircuits onto computer chips. The excimer laser mixes argon and fluoride gases, "exciting" them with electricity into a higher energy state and releasing powerful, ultraviolet light energy at a wavelength of 193nm (nanometers). Through a series of computer-controlled mirrors and prisms in the laser machine, the light is focused to emit an intensified beam powerful enough to vaporize (or "ablate") tissue. The excimer laser can reshape a cornea or, for that matter, etch a computer chip. Because the excimer laser is a cool laser, it can vaporize tissue while leaving the surrounding tissue undisturbed.

Like the word laser, LASIK is another acronym—laser-assisted in situ keratomileusis. *In situ* is Latin for "in the natural tissue" (not "in a test tube"). Keratomileusis is Greek—*kerato* means "cornea," and *mileusis* means "shaving or sculpting." During the first part of LASIK, a femtosecond laser or a microkeratome—a surgical, shaving instrument—makes an extremely fine incision in the cornea to create a corneal flap, which is lifted up and folded out of the way. During the second part of the procedure, the excimer laser reshapes the corneal tissue beneath the flap in-situ—in its natural state. The excimer laser is extremely precise, and, if programmed to remove 36μ (microns) of tissue to correct your vision, it will do exactly that. The corneal flap is then smoothed down over the newly ablated cornea, and the procedure is over.

PRK stands for photorefractive keratectomy. Photorefractive refers to the photons of light energy that are emitted by the excimer laser, whose beam removes a thin layer of corneal tissue to correct your refraction (keratectomy, like tonsillectomy). LASIK differs from PRK in that tissue is removed from under the flap in LASIK, while in PRK, tissue is removed from the surface of the cornea, making a flap unnecessary. During LASIK surgery, the flap is smoothed back in place, leaving the surface almost entirely untouched. The thin, U-shaped seam of the flap heals quickly, usually overnight, resulting in quicker healing and vision recovery. PRK surgery requires several days to a week or more for the surface epithelial layer of the cornea to completely regenerate. The visual results of LASIK and PRK are comparable.

Even though the vast majority of ophthalmologists advise LASIK for most patients, some patients have corneas that are not suitable for the creation of a flap. For those patients, PRK, or a newer hybrid procedure, LASEK, is generally recommended and gives excellent results.

LASEK stands for laser sub-epithelial keratomileusis. It combines aspects of both LASIK and PRK. In the first part of LASEK, a mild alcohol solution is used to loosen the epithelium, the delicate surface layer of the cornea. Once loosened, this gossamer-thin flap is brushed aside as one sheet of tissue. The laser treatment, the second part of LASEK, is then performed to correct the refractive error. The laser beam part of the procedure is identical to that of LASIK and PRK. After the ablation is completed, the epithelium is brushed back over the cornea into its original position. A soft contact lens that acts as a Band-Aid is placed on the cornea and remains there until the surface is healed—usually in less than a week.

Although a flap is created in both LASIK and LASEK, the LASEK flap heals more slowly than the LASIK flap. The weak alcohol solution used to loosen the epithelial layer of the LASEK cornea leaves the delicate cells damaged, so that new cells have to repopulate the flap just as new cells must grow over the surface of the cornea in PRK. The thicker LASIK flap carries with it undamaged epithelium resulting in faster healing. A new microkeratome, capable of creating an epithelial flap without the potentially damaging effects of alcohol, promises to speed healing in LASEK. Since the epithelial flap is created with a microkeratome, similar to that used in LASIK, the procedure is now called epi-LASIK, where "epi" means "on the surface." This is gradually replacing the classic LASEK, which uses alcohol to remove the surface epithelium. To take this a step further, PRK, LASEK and epi-LASIK now fall under the umbrella term, "Surface Ablation," as opposed to LASIK, where the excimer laser works under the surface.

The final results of LASIK and Surface Ablation (PRK, LASEK, and epi-LASIK) are comparable, though the amount of time required for healing varies. Your eye doctor can advise you which technique is best for you. With the help of this book, you should better understand your doctor's advice.

2

Eye Basics

To understand how LVC (laser vision correction) works, it is important to know how the eye functions. In this section, we will explore the reasons why approximately half the population on earth requires some form of vision correction.

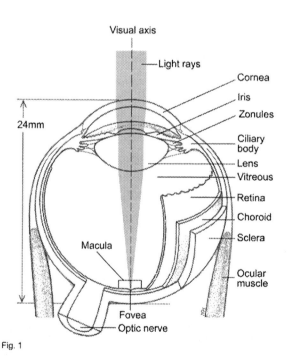

Fig. 1

Fig 1. The parts of the eye—light rays are focused to a sharp point on the retina, indicating no refractive error.

Actually, the eye doesn't see, the brain does. The eye admits rays of light and focuses that light into a perfect point on the retina—the thin membrane of rods and cones at the back of the eye (see figure 1). These photoreceptors then convert that light into nerve impulses that travel through the optic nerve to the brain.

Light enters the eye through the pupil—the black, round opening in the center of the iris—the colored part of the eye. The pupil opens (dilates) in dim light to admit more light. In brighter light, the pupil gets smaller (constricts) to limit the amount of light entering the eye. The iris controls the pupil and determines the color of your eye. A heavily pigmented iris results in a brown eye, while a lightly pigmented iris results in a blue or gray eye. The iris is surrounded by the sclera—the tough, white, outer wall of the eye. Although the iris is the most noticeable part of your eye, our LVC discussion focuses on the cornea—the transparent, dome-shaped front part of the eye.

Cornea Anatomy

The cornea is about the size and thickness of a dime, about one-half inch in diameter and 500μ–600μ (microns) thick in the center (a micron is one-millionth of a meter). Despite its small size, the cornea is a complex body part composed of five different layers, each one important in LVC (see figure 2).

Epithelium—the first or outer layer of the cornea's five layers is a clear, thin membrane, which acts as a barrier to microorganisms. The epithelium has a remarkable ability to regenerate—a small scratch from a foreign body often heals overnight while a bigger "scratch" from PRK may take 4–7 days. The epithelium is 30μ –50μ thick.

Bowman's membrane—the second layer of the cornea, made up of collagen fibrils, acts as a shield against trauma and infection, and is about 12μ–14μ thick. During all three forms of Surface Ablation, the epithelium is removed, leaving a smooth, glistening Bowman's membrane. This membrane is the first structure removed by the excimer laser during ablation, the stroma is the second.

Layers of cornea

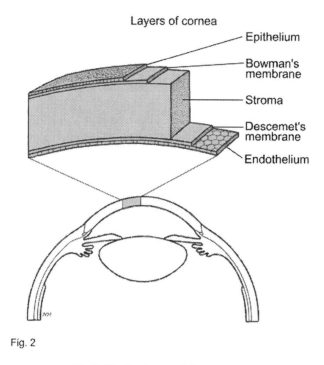

Fig. 2

Fig 2. The five layers of the cornea.

Stroma—the densest part of the cornea, is about 90% of the cornea's thickness. The stroma, consisting of lamellae—or layers of collagen fibers stacked in transparent, horizontal tiers—filters in light rays. The stroma is about 400μ–450μ thick.

Descemet's membrane—approximately 10μ–12μ thick, supports the lower corneal layers and acts as a dam to prevent the aqueous fluid inside the eye from seeping into the stroma and causing the stroma to swell and cloud.

Endothelium—the fifth and final layer of the cornea is one cell thick, and together with Descemet's membrane, helps keep the cornea relatively dehydrated, a state vital to the cornea's transparency. The endothelium features a metabolic pumping action that removes aqueous fluid from the cornea, preventing it from becoming cloudy. This pumping action helps the LASIK flap adhere to the stroma after being smoothed back into place. The endothelium is about 4μ–6μ thick.

Cornea and Vision

The curvature of the cornea and the length of your eye from front to back (the "axial" length) determine whether you need corrective lenses to see clearly. An overly curved, or "steep," cornea will make an average-length eye nearsighted or myopic, while a weakly curved, or "flat," cornea will result in a farsighted or hyperopic eye. Similarly, a long eye makes an average-curved cornea into a myopic or nearsighted eye, while a short eye results in a hyperopic or farsighted eye. A perfect balance between the cornea and the axial length means glasses are not required.

The cornea is one of two transparent tissues that determine your vision. The other, the crystalline lens—also clear and somewhat elastic—sits just behind the iris and helps the cornea focus light onto your retina. The muscular ciliary body is also behind the iris and regulates the shape of the lens by thousands of strands called zonules. When we focus our eyes, these muscles and zonules, much like the strings on a marionette, automatically control the shape of the crystalline lens, relaxing it to make it thin for distance vision or contracting to make it thicker for near vision. Two-thirds of the eye's focusing power comes from the cornea and one-third from the crystalline lens. Beginning as early as age twenty, the crystalline lens gradually loses its elasticity until, after age forty, it cannot change shape enough to bring close objects such as newspapers or menus into focus. The result is a common, virtually universal condition known as presbyopia (Latin for "old sight") and is easily corrected by reading glasses. CK—conductive keratoplasty—is a newer, non-laser alternative to reading glasses. For patients over forty who are having LVC, some reading vision can be preserved by sacrificing a small amount of distance vision in one eye with a special technique called monovision, (discussed in detail in Chapter Ten).

In summary, the pupil determines the amount of light entering the eye, the cornea bends or refracts that light, and the lens helps to focus that light.

However, there's more to the story. The back part of the eye is lined with the retina, a thin membrane that converts light into an electric impulse, which is then sent to the brain via the optic nerve. Light travels to the retina through the vitreous—the clear, jelly-like substance that fills the back cavity of the eye. Once the retina transforms the light and sends it to the brain, the brain sees what the eye transmits. All the different parts of the eye working together "take the picture," but the brain "develops the picture."

The macula, an area one-eighth inch wide near the optic nerve, is the most important part of the retina. The macula, particularly the fovea—a tiny pit at its center—is responsible for most of our clear, central vision. The remainder of the retina provides our less distinct but crucial peripheral vision. The macula—the "bull's-eye of the retina"—gives us detail.

Vision is created by the journey of light through the eye to the brain. Vision errors result from imperfections in that journey. Glasses, contact lenses, and refractive surgery all attempt to correct vision errors.

Vision Errors

For vision to be clear without glasses or contacts, at least three structures of the eye must work in perfect unison: the cornea, the crystalline lens, and the retina. The main function of the cornea and the crystalline lens is to bend light from objects to a pinpoint focus on the macula—the critical, central part of the retina. This exact focus gives us sharp, clear vision. Whether light rays enter the eye parallel, as they do from distant objects, or nonparallel (divergent), as they do from near objects such as this book, the cornea and crystalline lens must refract them correctly so that the light rays focus precisely on the retina.

Vision errors occur when there are discrepancies among the focusing power of the cornea, the lens, or both and the eye's axial length—the distance from the cornea to the retina. Four types of vision errors can result: presbyopia, myopia, hyperopia, and astigmatism. Most of us, unfortunately, will have at least two of these errors during our lives. Presbyopia ("old eyes") is a virtually universal condition that affects everyone who lives past age forty. It is a natural part of aging and is the only vision error that is almost totally due to changes in the crystalline lens, rather than the cornea. With age the lens becomes slightly compacted and loses its flexibility. This loss of flexibility begins around age twenty, but it is not until age forty that the lens is no longer able to change shape to focus on near objects. At some point during middle age, a menu or a newspaper gradually must be held more and more at arm's length to be readable, and eventually your arms won't be long enough. Reading glasses, often from the drug store, or bifocal contact lenses will bring instant relief. Monovision, with one eye modified for near vision, and one eye modified for distance vision, is an LVC option available for presbyopia.

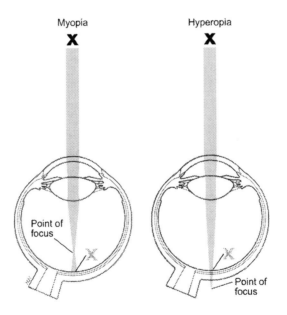

Fig. 3

Fig 3. In myopia, light rays focus on a point in front of, rather than on, the retina. In hyperopia, light rays focus behind the retina. The rays that fall on the retina are unfocused resulting in blurred vision.

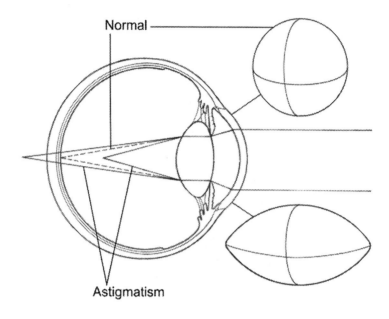

Fig. 4

Fig 4. Astigmatism occurs when light rays are focused into two
distinct points.

The three other types of vision errors—myopia, hyperopia, and astigmatism—are cornea-related and are refractive errors. In many cases, these conditions can be cured by LVC. More than half of the human race suffers from refractive errors.

Myopia (from the Greek "shut eyes" refers to squinting by near-sighted people to see better through a "pinhole") is also known as nearsightedness and occurs when you can see near objects but distant objects are blurry. The condition occurs when the curvature of the cornea is too steep or the axial length of the eye is too long. Instead of falling onto a sharp focus point on the retina, light is overly focused and falls in front of the retina (see figure 3). LVC surgery flattens the overly steep curvature of the cornea so the light from distant objects hits the pinpoint center of the macula, focusing objects sharply and clearly.

Hyperopia or farsightedness is the opposite condition. Because the curvature of the cornea is too flat or the axial length of the eye is too short, light is focused behind the retina. Unlike myopia, a condition in which blurred distance vision is noticeable early in life, hyperopia is often "silent," revealing signs of near and distant blurred vision only as we age. This occurs because the elastic, natural crystalline lens of a young hyperope thickens in response to focusing muscles in the ciliary body, providing 20/20 vision despite a fair amount of hyperopia. With age, this "latent" hyperopia becomes too much for our aging eye muscles to "self-correct," resulting in blurred vision. Vision surgery does not elongate or shorten the eye, but the effect of making the front surface of the eye flatter or steeper results in light reaching the retina on target.

The fourth refractive error is astigmatism (see figure 4). Presbyopia is the aging of the crystalline lens, and myopia or hyperopia is an imbalance between the curvature, or power, of the cornea and the length of the eye. Astigmatism has nothing to do with axial length. The word astigmatism comes from the Greek, *a* (without) and *stigma* (point). Light passes through the cornea to two points of focus. Astigmatism is caused by a corneal curvature that is oval-shaped rather than perfectly round. A non-astigmatic or spherical cornea is shaped like a baseball and bends light uniformly. An astigmatic cornea is football-shaped, focusing light to one point on the long axis of the "football" and to a second point on the short axis. These two points can straddle the retina, one behind and one in front, or one point can land on the retina, while the other point can fall either in front of the retina or behind it. To achieve clear vision, eyeglasses or contact lenses fuse the two points of light and move that single point onto the retina. Although astigmatism blurs both near and far vision, it is corrected by the excimer laser in much the same way as is myopia or hyperopia, although slightly less accurately. Patients usually have astigmatism combined with myopia or hyperopia, and over half of patients with these two refractive errors have some degree of astigmatism. Pure astigmatism is very rare.

LVC and the Cornea—A Brief Overview

Laser Vision Correction (LVC) is accomplished by removing, or "ablating," a thin layer of the stroma—the thickest part of the cornea and the part that gives it shape and curvature. For a nearsighted treatment, approximately 12μ of stromal tissue removal equals a correction of about one diopter (D) of myopia and takes about eight seconds (or forty-eight pulses of the excimer laser). These figures change slightly depending on manufacturer and model of the excimer laser used. The duration of the ablation portion of surgery depends on your eyeglass prescription and whether you are nearsighted or farsighted—the higher the correction, the longer the duration of laser treatment. Myopic ablations generally take less time than hyperopic ablations. Unlike the superficial epithelium, which regenerates after a corneal scratch or after PRK, the stroma does not regenerate, so vision correction will generally last many years, often for the rest of your life. Corneal thickness varies from person to person and from eye to eye, even in the same patient. While only a small portion of the upper layer of the stroma is ablated during LVC, at least 250μ of intact stroma must remain for the health and integrity of the cornea. Corneal thickness is measured during the eye examination, and if the cornea is not thick enough for LASIK, then PRK or another form of Surface Ablation would be more suitable because there is no stromal flap created in these two procedures.

In nearsighted patients, the laser flattens the center of the cornea. The treatment zone, the area of the cornea treated by the laser ablation, is in the center of the cornea and gradually tapers to the periphery. One of the lessons learned from the early days of LVC is to make the treatment zone as wide as, or wider than, the size of the pupil in dim light to minimize the occurrence of glare, halos, and star bursts.

In farsighted patients, the center of the cornea must be made steeper by removing tissue in a donut-shaped pattern on the cornea, leaving the center relatively untouched. The center bulges forward, the curvature increases, and the hyperopia is corrected. A good analogy would be to picture you and your closest five friends standing in a circle on a waterbed—the center of the bed would bulge upward.

Astigmatism, caused by an oval-shaped cornea, is a combination of steepness in one direction and flatness in another. Similarly, the excimer laser treatment flattens and steepens accordingly, resulting in a spherical cornea.

Vision Correction

We live in the golden age of vision correction. We have a multitude of vision corrective devices and surgical procedures and equipment that examine every component of the eye in depth. The goal of any excimer laser ablation and treatment is to correct your vision and your refractive error. In order to best understand that correction, let's look at how vision is measured so you can better understand your own vision prescription.

3

The Eye Examination

Your Prescription

Do you have 20/20 eyesight? This common standard is what most people associate with normal vision. What does it take to reach 20/20? Do you need a strong prescription? Do you need a weak prescription? Are your eyeglasses thick or thin? Can you cross the street without your glasses or must you wear them to see a foot in front of you? You may be surprised to know that, although you may be concerned if your eyeglass prescription changes from mild to moderate, this has little significance to an ophthalmologist, whose main concern is that your best corrected visual acuity (BCVA) remains 20/20. Maintaining a patient's BCVA is a major goal of LVC.

If a patient with moderate myopia, correctable with glasses to 20/20, has LVC and remains slightly nearsighted, he or she will be disappointed, but if the BCVA remains 20/20 with a mild eyeglass correction, the eye is considered healthy. There may be a slight loss of BCVA when correcting higher levels of refractive errors, but in most cases the trade off is worth it and the patient, free from glasses, is happy. Except for extremely high prescriptions, the 20/20 level of vision is more representative of eye health than the level of the refractive error.

Reading the Chart

During an eye examination, we look at a chart with lines of letters, numbers, or symbols that progressively decrease in size as we read down the chart. This is known as the Snellen eye chart, devised by

Dutch ophthalmologist Hermann Snellen in 1862 to measure visual acuity ("acuity" from the Latin, *acuitas* for sharpness). Legend has it that Snellen's examining room was about twenty feet long and, using his assistant who had normal vision, Snellen selected the lowest line of letters his assistant could barely read, and designated that line as "20/20." The patient stands twenty feet—the standard measuring distance—away from the chart and reads the line marked 20/20 (see figure 5). Glasses or contacts are used to correct your vision to your BCVA—Best Corrected Visual Acuity. The most common "normal" BCVA is 20/20, but some patients have a BCVA of 20/10, while for others, it is 20/30. The measurement of visual acuity is not very scientific, because one patient might be able to easily read the 20/20 line while another will need coaxing and encouragement from the eye doctor to read the 20/20 line. Both patients, however, have 20/20 vision.

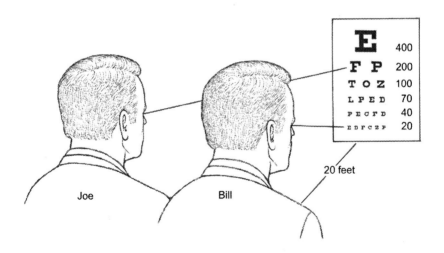

Fig. 5

Fig 5. From 20 feet away, Bill can see the small letters on line 20, while Joe can see only large letters on line 200. Bill has 20/20 vision; Joe has 20/200 vision. (By definition, with 20/20 vision, Bill can see line 20 from 20 feet, and can also see line 200 from 200 feet.)

Visual acuity of 20/40 means that at twenty feet, you can read down only to the 20/40 line, which features larger type. The second number determines the line you can read, and the higher the number, the worse your visual acuity. Some people have 20/15 or even 20/10 visual acuity. On the other hand, if you have best corrected visual acuity of 20/200, you may be considered legally blind in most states. If you are 20/30 or 20/40, uncorrected, you still may be able to drive without glasses.

The Eyeglass Prescription

Having visual acuity less than 20/20 doesn't always mean you need glasses. Many people with 20/25 or 20/30 vision are unaffected by a slight blur for long distance. Once vision reaches 20/40 or worse, part-time or full-time glasses or contact lenses are usually needed. The aim of corrective lenses is to achieve BCVA, whether that is 20/20, 20/25, or 20/15.

Eyeglass prescriptions are written in diopters (D), a unit of measurement of the refracting power of the lens, similar to measuring length in feet and weight in pounds. In general, prescriptions increase or decrease in one-fourth diopter increments, and the higher the number, the stronger the lens.

Consider a typical, non-astigmatic myopic prescription:

O.D. −2.50

O.S. −2.00

O.D. (*oculus dexter* in Latin) is the abbreviation for the right eye, and O.S. (*oculus sinister*) is the abbreviation for the left eye. The numbers, −2.50 and −2.00 respectively, are followed by D, (e.g., −2.50 D). D stands for diopters. Eye doctors would call this patient a 2-diopter myope.

The prescription used in our example would be that of a low to moderate myope, a range that includes anyone falling into the prescription power category of −1.00 D to approximately −6.00 D. If your prescription features numbers preceded by a (+) plus sign instead of a (−)

minus sign, you are a hyperope. Although there are many myopes with prescriptions stronger than 3D, most hyperopes are less than 3D. LVC for hyperopes is usually more successful in patients below 3 or 4 D. Whether you are a myope or hyperope, if you are over the age of forty-five, your eyeglass prescription will also have an age-appropriate "add." This addition is extra power that is added to your eyeglass lens as either a separate reading glass or as part of a bifocal to help you read small print. A typical add power for a forty-five-year-old is +1.50, so if your eye distance prescription is –4.00 D, you would need –2.50 D power in the bifocal portion of your glasses [(–4.00) + (+1.50) = –2.50 D]. If you wear contacts, you could use +1.50 "magnifiers" from the drugstore to wear over your contacts. If you are a forty-five-year-old +3.00 D hyperope, you would need a total power of + 4.50 D in reading glasses, or in the bifocal, in order to read [(+3.00) + (+1.50) = +4.50]. The contact lens wearer, whether a hyperope or a myope, would still use the same +1.50 D drug store reading glasses over the contacts.

Astigmatism

Deciphering your astigmatism prescription is a little trickier. A typical astigmatism prescription for someone's right eye has three parts:

O.D. –2.50 D + 1.00 D x 90

The –2.50 diopters is technically called the "sphere" and refers to the overall shape or curvature of the cornea. If the cornea in this example were round instead of oval or football-shaped, the patient would have no astigmatism and be a –2.50 myope. The second and third numbers refer to the astigmatism, indicating how much the cornea resembles a football, and in what direction the football is resting—either the fat part on the ground, the pointy tip on the ground, or somewhere in between. In our example, "+1.00 D x 90" means that the cornea is more steeply curved in the vertical direction (meridian) than the horizontal direction, the difference being one diopter between the two meridians. In eyeglass prescriptions, the "+1.00" is called the "cylinder" and the "x" is the axis. Non-astigmatic corneas are spherical and have no difference in curvature between the two meridians.

A prescription for astigmatism can be written in plus cylinder form or in minus cylinder form—both will mean the same thing. For example, the prescription –2.50 D +1.00 D x 90 could be written using a minus sign before the cylinder and would be –1.50 D –1.00 D x 180. The absolute value of the cylinder, +1.00 D, is added to the sphere, –2.50 D, [–2.50 D + (+1.00 D) = –1.50 D] and the axis is changed ninety degrees. If you are considering LVC, it is helpful to understand the concepts behind your prescription. Most prescriptions can now be corrected by LVC or by newer methods to be discussed later.

Your Eye Exam

Though LVC is not appropriate for everyone, a thorough eye exam, the foundation of all refractive surgery, will determine if you are a good candidate. Even though you "pass" this exam, tests done specifically for LVC will either confirm or disqualify you as a candidate for LVC.

Patient History

The first step of any eye health exam is reviewing the patient's history. Your ophthalmologist will ask you about both your overall health and your eye health. It is important to be completely honest. Most candidates for refractive surgery are twenty-five to fifty-five years old and healthy, but some seemingly common diseases can disqualify you as a candidate. Autoimmune problems, such as rheumatoid arthritis and ulcerative colitis, can be associated with rare but serious cornea problems, so LVC may not be appropriate. Eye disease, such as lazy eye from childhood (amblyopia), glaucoma (elevated pressure in the eye), severe dry eye, and retinal detachment may all affect vision adversely, causing rare complications following LVC surgery. Pregnancy, lactation, certain medications—such as Accutane for acne, Imitrex for migraines and amiodarone for heart problems—are usually contraindications for LVC.

A complete history includes questions about lifestyle, work, leisure activities, and other vision tasks that you perform most often. If you are considering LVC, your ophthalmologist will also ask about your motivation for the surgery to determine whether you have realistic expectations. Every patient who elects to have LVC should expect to wear glasses for some tasks, such as driving at night or sitting in the back of a theater. Often, even for these activities, glasses may not be necessary, but anticipating the need for glasses for some activities and having realistic expectations can be the difference between a satisfied patient and a disappointed one.

Visual Acuity and Refraction

The next step in the eye exam is the refraction to determine your best corrected visual acuity. Your BCVA should be 20/40 or better—normal vision for most people. If your BCVA is abnormal, the eye exam will uncover the reason, such as glaucoma, cataracts, corneal or retinal disease. For the excimer laser to accurately correct your vision, your refraction must be precisely measured, more so than when you are fitted with glasses or contact lenses. Your eye doctor may measure your refraction in several ways.

The refraction usually will start with the auto-refractor (short for automated refractor)—a computerized device that uses infrared light to measure your refractive error. In the examining room, the auto-refractor measurement is entered into the phoropter, a butterfly-like device containing hundreds of lenses that is mounted on a swing arm. The phoropter is positioned in front of your eyes, and as you look through it at lines on the Snellen chart, your doctor will find the combination of lenses that gives you your BCVA. Because the reading from the auto-refractor is not always 100% accurate, your eye doctor may still ask, "Which is better, one or two?" While the resulting "manifest" refraction is fairly accurate, dilating your pupils with eye drops to temporarily weaken your focusing ability may provide an even greater degree of accuracy. Unbeknownst to you, your ciliary muscles can spontaneously focus and relax your crystalline lens, significantly altering your refraction. Ciliary muscle contraction can falsely increase the degree of myopia, making you seem more nearsighted or less farsighted than you really are. To exclude this factor from your final refraction and avoid reshaping your cornea for a greater refractive error than is actually present, your ophthalmologist will often perform a cycloplegic refraction—a refraction using cycloplegic or focus-weakening eye drops. Cyclogyl or Mydriacyl, the eye drops used in the cycloplegic or "wet" refraction, take about 20–30 minutes to work. Your eye doctor will then repeat the same "dry" refraction exam you had prior to the drops. A cygloplegic refraction can be more accurate than a dry, manifest refraction. The younger you are, the stronger and more interfering your focusing muscles are, and the more your eye doctor may rely on the cycloplegic refraction. Because contact lenses can change the shape of your cornea and alter your refraction, your eye doctor may ask you to stop wearing your lenses for a period of time—usually a week or two for soft contact lenses, and two or more weeks for gas permeable contacts.

External Examination

In this part of the eye examination, your eye doctor will use the slit lamp as well as a penlight, a small flashlight the size of a pen, to check your eyelids for any sign of infection or inflammation, your pupils for abnormalities, and the alignment of your eyes.

Blepharitis, a common inflammatory disorder of the lids caused by excessive oil production and flaking, must be eliminated before surgery because bacteria can live and breed in the crust and debris on the lids. Treatment is simple and usually entails using hot compresses, followed by warm water and baby shampoo to cleanse the lids.

The eye doctor also checks your pupils, alternately shining the light in one eye and then the other. Each pupil should equally and quickly contract in response to light. Examining the position of your eyes and function of your eye muscles occurs next. By covering one eye and then the other as you read the Snellen chart, the ophthalmologist will be able to tell if your eyes are working together, or if one eye tends to drift out or cross in. Minor discrepancies in the alignment and straightness of your eyes are common, and should be detected before surgery. The degree to which your eyes cross or wander can be influenced by your refractive error. Refractive surgery, which changes your refractive error, may unmask eye muscle imbalance and potentially can result in double vision.

Slit Lamp

The slit lamp, a "biomicroscope," is the machine on which you rest your chin and press your forehead against a headrest as your ophthalmologist looks through two eyepieces that resemble binoculars. The slit lamp is a central component of the eye exam. By focusing and moving a vertical, slit beam of light into the patient's eyes, the eye doctor gets a magnified stereoscopic view of the front portion of the eye—the cornea, iris, and crystalline lens—collectively called the anterior segment of the eye.

For refractive surgery, the cornea is of greatest concern because that is the site of surgery. Previous conditions, such as ocular herpes, bacterial infections, and foreign bodies can leave scar tissue and thinned areas of the cornea. Of main concern for LASIK is the detection of basement membrane dystrophy (BMD). This condition is seen under the slit lamp as white whirls and swirls on the surface of the cornea, representing areas where the surface epithelium does not fully adhere to the rest of the cornea. During the creation of the corneal flap in LASIK, poorly adherent areas of surface epithelium may be loosened and abraded by the microkeratome, resulting in an abrasion. Although healing can take longer and complications are more likely, especially with a large abrasion, the final outcome is still quite good. The immediate treatment consists of a bandage soft contact lens worn until the cornea heals, usually overnight. Surface Ablation or Intralasik, in which the LASIK flap is made with a laser instead of a microkeratome (discussed in Chapter Nine) may be more suitable for patients with basement membrane dystrophy to avoid the potential for an epithelial abrasion.

Tonometer

Tonometry, performed while you are still at the slit lamp, is a measurement of your intraocular pressure (IOP) with a tonometer, a probe-like device attached to the slit lamp. The measurement of your IOP is part of any thorough eye exam. Elevated IOP may indicate glaucoma, which usually consists of a triad of elevated IOP, optic nerve damage, and loss of areas within your field of vision. IOP alone is not the sole criteria for determining glaucoma because optic nerve damage, the main criterion for diagnosing glaucoma, may be present in the absences of elevated IOP. A recent, extensive study of glaucoma patients found that a thin cornea may give falsely low values for IOP, making it possible to overlook glaucoma. A thin cornea may also make your eye more susceptible to optic nerve damage from elevated IOP than a thick cornea would. Because LVC thins your cornea, it is important to have a comprehensive glaucoma test before LVC.

Retina Exam

While you are still seated, your ophthalmologist will examine the back of your eye—the retina. This is done with a small handheld lens, either at the slit lamp or with an indirect ophthalmoscope—a binocular-like device worn on a headband around the forehead. Frequently, your eye doctor may use both methods to look at your entire retina and optic nerve. The retinal exam is usually performed when your eyes are dilated because the peripheral portions of your retina can be seen only when your pupils are fully dilated. A careful examination of the retina is an important part of your general eye exam, especially if you are nearsighted. Nearsighted patients have a greater chance of having tiny tears or holes in the retina, which, in rare cases, can lead to a detached retina. If detected early, a simple retina tear can be easily treated with a laser (different from the one that is used in LVC) and, in most cases, prevents the more serious detached retina.

LVC Exam

The testing procedures described above are all components of a general eye exam. If you are being evaluated for vision correction surgery, your ophthalmologist will perform further tests to see if you are a good candidate and if so, which LVC procedure would be best suited to your eye and your needs.

Pupilography

The size of your pupil in the dark is an important measurement used to determine whether you are a good candidate for LVC. Although less important today with improved excimer lasers, size matters when it comes to the pupil because of the treatment zone, the circular area on your cornea that will be ablated. If the size of your pupil in the dark is significantly larger than the treatment zone, light that hits the edge of the treatment zone will scatter into your eye and may cause you to see halos and starbursts at night when your pupil is larger. To measure pupils when they are at their most dilated, the eye doctor darkens the exam room and uses a pupilometer or other measuring device. Although the importance of pupil size on successful LVC is somewhat controversial, very large pupils, especially at higher prescriptions, may rule out surgery to avoid the possibility of disabling glare disturbances. However, most modern lasers can be set to accommodate a larger pupil, making it is less likely that pupil size will disqualify you from LVC. Custom ablation, discussed in depth later, minimizes annoying halos or starbursts and may be a good choice for patients with large pupils. Your eye doctor will need to provide guidance.

Keratometer

The keratometer is an instrument that measures the cornea's curvature. This measurement is critical for several reasons. The microkeratome used in LASIK has several attachments, or rings, that are selected by your ophthalmologist to create the proper size flap. Corneal curvature largely determines this microkeratome setting, emphasizing the importance of the keratometer measurement. Corneal curvature may also initially disqualify you from having LVC. LVC flattens the myope's cornea and steepens the hyperope's. Knowing your corneal curvature and the change induced by the laser treatment will give your eye doctor an estimate of the curvature that will remain following the surgery. Even though your vision may improve to 20/20, the quality of vision may not be optimal if your cornea is made too flat or too steep in an attempt to correct your refractive error. LVC may be ill-advised for a myope with a too-flat cornea or a hyperope with a too-steep cornea.

Corneal Pachymetry

The ultrasound pachymeter is a small box that generates radar-like sound waves to record the thickness of your cornea. A cord attached to the box terminates in an ultrasound probe that gently touches the surface of the cornea and records its thickness. LVC removes corneal tissue, and, because the cornea must be sufficiently thick for eye health after LVC, it is critical to know the thickness before and after LVC. The remaining, healthy "corneal bed" should be at least 250μ thick. During LVC, the excimer laser removes an average of 12μ of tissue to correct each diopter of myopia. If a –5.00 diopter myope has a corneal thickness of 590μ, the calculations might be: 590μ – 60μ (5 x 12 = 60) – 160μ flap (flap thickness of LASIK which no longer contributes to the strength of the cornea) = 590 – 220 = 370μ—well above the 250μ minimum. A –5.00 myope with a corneal thickness of 450μ has a cornea that would be too thin for LASIK (450 – 160 – 60 = 230),—below the 250μ minimum, but might be fine for PRK, which does not require a flap. There is some controversy among eye surgeons whether PRK should even be done on anyone with a corneal thickness less than 480 or 490μ. More on this later.

Corneal pachymetry is especially important if you are nearsighted because the laser thins the center of the cornea. Farsighted vision requires the laser to remove tissue from the normally thicker outer cornea. Your eye doctor will calculate the predicted corneal thickness if LASIK is considered. If your cornea is too thin for LASIK, then PRK, LASEK, or epi-LASIK is usually the better choice.

Corneal Topography

Corneal topography (CT) is a computerized, color, topographical map of the cornea, similar to geological maps of mountains and valleys. Corneal topography provides a color-coded graphic representation of the corneal surface and reveals abnormalities, irregularities, or aberrations that would make laser surgery inadvisable. CT is especially important in diagnosing early forms of keratoconus (KC), a corneal disease in which the cornea becomes thin and extremely steepened or curved. In its early or "form fruste" stage, KC may have no signs or symptoms and often can be seen only on corneal topography. Conventional LVC requires a cornea with little or no irregularities. Wavefront customized LVC, the latest and most high-tech ophthalmic innovation to date, promises to correct many types of irregularities of the cornea, but KC, even in its early stages, is generally a contraindication even for LVC.

Wavefront Exam

Wavefront technology promises to give patients the best chance for improved vision, often better than the 20/20 made possible with glasses or contact lenses. Scientists in astronomy and physics developed wavefront technology to measure and reduce aberrations or imperfections in the optical systems of high-powered telescopes, mostly for military use. This technology was adapted to measure imperfections in the eye in the hope of creating supernormal vision. Credit goes to Johannes Hartman, Roland Shack, and Josef Bille for using wavefront technology to measure the total imperfections of the human eye, rather than just the refractive error.

The eye's wavefront is measured with a computerized instrument called an aberrometer, which first sends infrared light into your eye. The aberrometer then analyzes the wavefront of light reflected off the retina as it passes through the entire optical system (especially the crystalline lens and cornea).

If the patient's optical system has perfect refracting surfaces, the wavefront exits out through the eye in a regular pattern. Any aberrations in the shape or on the surface of the cornea or other parts of the eye will result in an irregular wavefront.

In a custom wavefront LASIK treatment, the aberrometer downloads the wavefront onto an external hard drive, which then programs the excimer laser. The laser, guided by the wavefront program, attempts to correct not only your refractive error, but also any and all aberrations in the cornea. Fewer aberrations mean better vision.

The aberrometer measures several types of aberrations. "Low order" aberrations are the most common and include myopia, hyperopia, and astigmatism. Higher order aberrations, such as "coma" and "trefoil," can affect the quality of vision. While not yet a reality, correction of all higher order aberrations in customized wavefront LASIK treatment may someday be possible, offering patients the chance for supernormal vision.

Post Exam

By now, you've had the longest, most meticulous eye exam of your life. The best ophthalmologist for performing surgery on your eyes is one who is detail-oriented and thorough. Even though today's technology can give your ophthalmologist an unprecedented level of data, medicine is not only about machines. It is also about knowledge, training, and skilled individuals providing the best care possible. Your eye doctor will use the data collected during a thorough LVC eye exam to determine whether you can have LVC and if so, which surgical procedure is best for you.

You should feel comfortable asking questions. After the exam, you should have answers to at least six questions:

1. Is laser surgery suitable for you?

2. What procedure is best for you—LASIK or Surface Ablation?

3. What are the chances of operative or postoperative complications?

4. How long will the healing process take?

5. What are the chances for 20/40 vision or for 20/20 vision?

6. Will you still need to wear glasses part-time?

4

Laser Vision Correction: LASIK, PRK, LASEK, and Epi-LASIK

The golden age of vision correction promises to improve. Until the 1950s, patients needing vision correction settled for spectacles. In the 1950s, contact lenses became available, but there was only one choice—hard lenses—with associated comfort problems. In the 1970s, soft contact lenses gave millions of patients relief from the discomfort of hard lenses, ushering in a revolution in contact lenses. A smorgasbord of soft lens choices evolved, from daily disposable, toric (correcting astigmatism), and continuous overnight wear to bifocal and multifocal lenses. Colored lenses can change brown eyes to blue, blue eyes to green, and every color in between. For those patients with too much astigmatism for soft lenses, the hard lens was replaced by a more comfortable gas-permeable lens that offered improved vision and comfort.

Now, the promise of regaining your natural eyesight, of being truly free of glasses or contact lenses, of literally turning back the clock to the days before you had to wear any type of corrective lenses, is here. Two types of procedures make that possible: LASIK and Surface Ablation (LASEK, PRK, and epi-LASIK). Other procedures may be suitable for some patients, but for most patients, Laser Vision Correction has propelled our golden age of vision correction to heights we could not have imagined as recently as ten years ago. A thorough exam or discussion with your doctor will determine if you are a candidate for this remarkable laser treatment.

LASIK (or laser-assisted in situ keratomilieusis) is the most commonly performed LVC in the world, accounting for more than 90% of LVC procedures. What makes LASIK so popular is the rapid improvement of vision when compared to other forms of LVC. No matter how strong your prescription is, the average LVC patient can usually pass a driver's vision test twenty-four hours after surgery, often even after only one hour. This quick, often miraculous recovery is due to the microkeratome—an instrument similar to a carpenter's plane. The surgeon places the microkeratome on the cornea after using numbing eye drops and, using a suction device to lock the microkeratome into place, creates a corneal flap (figure 6). This thin flap of corneal tissue is folded out of the way and the excimer laser removes a thin layer of corneal tissue to correct your vision—flattening your cornea if you are myopic, steepening your cornea if you are hyperopic, or rounding it out if you are astigmatic. The surgeon then smoothes down the flap, fitting it back exactly where it came from, like a piece in a jigsaw puzzle, over the ablated area. The corneal flap adheres to the rest of the cornea within minutes and the procedure is over.

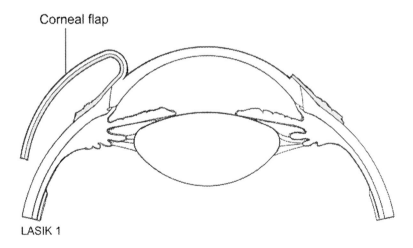

Corneal flap

LASIK 1

Fig. 6a

Fig 6a. The corneal flap consists of epithelium and stroma.

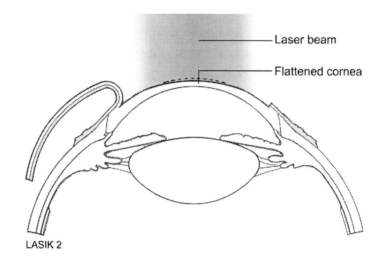

Fig. 6b

Fig 6b. The laser ablation.

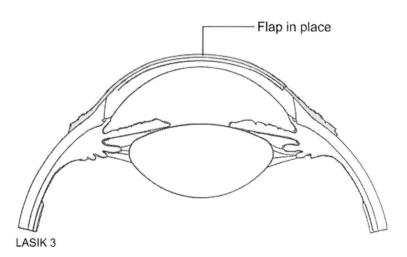

Fig. 6c

Fig 6c. The corneal flap is smoothed down into its original position.

In matter of a few hours, patients burdened for years with wearing glasses or contact lenses often achieve vision so clear that the first word out of their mouths is an incredulous, "Wow." Why does vision recover so quickly? The answer is that the corneal surface in the line of sight (visual axis) remains practically untouched. When the flap of corneal tissue is created, the U-shaped narrow seam is the only area of the cornea's surface that is disrupted. The surface and center of the cornea, the part through which you see, is untouched. Within a few hours or overnight, the seam, or "gutter," fills in with new cells that grow very rapidly across the seam. In the average patient, by the following morning the flap has adhered, the seam has healed, and that clock across the room is no longer the blur it was the day before.

The corneal flap also makes it easier to perform enhancements. If you did not achieve the level of vision you wanted, another laser treatment may be performed a few months or even years later. The surgeon carefully breaks the seal on the flap, lifting the flap once again as in the original procedure, and performs an additional laser ablation. Enhancements are usually very successful, but may not be advisable if your original, untreated cornea was thin.

If the rapidly healing corneal flap is largely responsible for the wow factor, it is also responsible for the majority of complications that can result from LASIK. The flap can be too thin, too thick, too small, irregular, incomplete, or "button-holed." It can develop wrinkles, folds, and striae—all of which can lead to delayed or poor healing or a poor visual result. Fortunately, these problems occur in less than 1% of LVC patients and can usually be treated successfully. Read more about complications in Chapter Seven.

PRK, or photorefractive keratectomy, preceded LASIK and was the first LVC operation to be widely used. Although it has been largely supplanted by LASIK, PRK is still preferable for many patients, especially for those for whom LASIK is unsuitable. Even for patients for whom LASIK is suitable, PRK is still a viable option.

During PRK, no corneal flap is created. The epithelium, the thin layer of cells on the surface of the cornea, is removed either by a preliminary laser ablation or by the use of a diluted alcohol solution that softens the epithelium, allowing it to be wiped away (see figures 7a and 7b). An Amoils brush, an electric toothbrush-like device is also commonly used to remove the surface epithelium. A well-defined, round defect or abrasion, wide enough for the laser treatment, remains on the surface of the cornea.

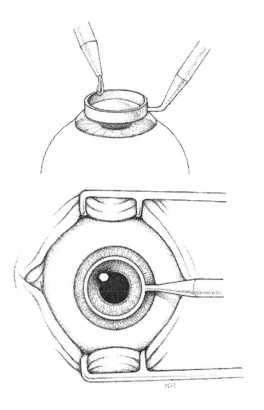

Fig. 7a

Fig 7a. Diluted alcohol is dropped into a "trephine" on the cornea to soften the surface epithelium.

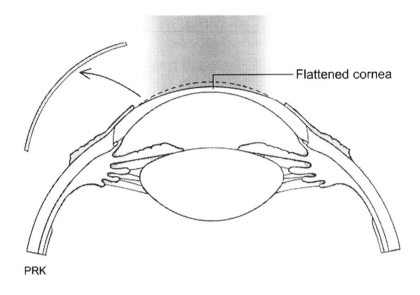

Fig. 7b

Fig 7b. During PRK, the epithelium is removed, and the laser
reshapes the cornea.

Once the epithelial tissue is removed, the laser treatment is identical
to that of LASIK and the results of LASIK and PRK are essentially the
same. PRK takes several days to a week or more to heal. Rather than a
thin, corneal flap seam left by LASIK that begins to heal in a few hours,
PRK requires healing of the entire surface defect. New epithelial cells
gradually grow across the cornea's surface, and cell by cell, the defect
fills in over several days. If you have ever scratched a cornea, you know
how painful it can be, but PRK pain is kept to a tolerable minimum
with eye drops and a bandage soft contact lens that is placed on the eye
at the end of the procedure and removed only after the cornea is
healed.

If PRK takes so much longer to heal than LASIK, why has there
been a resurgence of PRK? The answer is that most of the complications with LASIK result from the flap, which sometimes can be irregular, incomplete, wrinkled, or dislodged. Although flap problems occur

in less than 1% of LASIK procedures, the safety of the flapless PRK may be attractive for many patients seeking LVC. However, there is a trade-off in deciding on PRK rather than LASIK, and that trade-off is the possibility of haze. Within months and even up to a year after PRK, an inexplicable haze or cloudiness can develop in the cornea, reducing vision to varying degrees. The haze is thought to be created by substances secreted by regenerated corneal tissue. Anti-inflammatory drops may be used for several months after PRK to prevent haze. If haze develops, it is often self-limiting, clearing on its own or with anti-inflammatory drops used over several months. This main drawback of PRK is uncommon in myopes with a prescription below –6.00 D and uncommon in any hyperope. Haze is less common with modern lasers and can be all but prevented with medication.

LASEK, also known as laser sub-epithelial keratectomy, was developed by Italian ophthalmologist Massimo Camellin in 1999, and combines surgical attributes of both LASIK and PRK. During LASEK surgery, the surface epithelial tissue that is removed during PRK is preserved. Unlike LASIK, there is no true corneal flap. During LASEK and as in PRK, the surface epithelial layer of the cornea is loosened with a diluted solution of alcohol (see figure 7a), then brushed to one side and retained out of the way of the laser (see figure 8). After the excimer laser ablates corneal tissue, as in either PRK or LASIK, the epithelial tissue is gently smoothed back into place. This stage of the procedure is similar to the corneal flap created during LASIK, although the tissue in the LASEK flap is much thinner and more delicate, consisting of the 50μ epithelial layer only and no stroma. In fact, if the LASEK flap is incomplete or fragmented, it may be discarded, transforming the operation into a standard PRK.

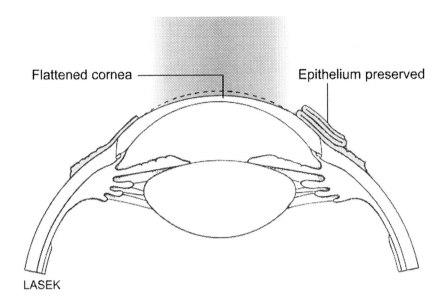

Flattened cornea   Epithelium preserved

LASEK

Fig. 8

Fig 8. The epithelial layer is folded off to one side; the laser ablation reshapes the cornea.

Ophthalmic surgeons debate whether the epithelial cells in the gossamer-thin flap are killed by the diluted alcohol solution and must completely regenerate or whether enough cells survive to grow across the cornea, thus accelerating healing. No conclusion has been drawn, but the trend now is to discard the epithelial flap and allow healing to take place as in routine PRK. The trend even carries over into epi-LASIK, where, despite the viability of the epithelial flap made without alcohol, the flap is still discarded. There is evidence, though still debate, that healing is faster with epi-LASIK than with PRK or LASEK. No matter which method is used, healing is usually complete within a week.

Another advantage of LASEK and especially epi-LASIK over PRK, besides the possible faster healing, is the chance of less haze. There is mounting and compelling evidence, still debatable among eye surgeons, that, especially at higher prescriptions, haze is less likely in LASEK and epi-LASIK. Although haze is less common than it was several years ago thanks to improvements in the excimer laser itself, the use of mitomycin C, a solution applied to the cornea immediately after the ablation, has reduced the possibility of haze even further.

Because of LASIK's more rapid healing and less discomfort, the majority of ophthalmologists, myself included, still prefer LASIK to Surface Ablation for their patients. Surface Ablation has increased in popularity among many eye surgeons due to the advent of the microkeratome for epi-LASIK and the use of new medication to ease discomfort.

LASIK is not possible or advisable for all patients for several reasons, chiefly relating to corneal thickness and integrity. Although the corneal flap created during LASIK adheres to the rest of the cornea during the healing process, it no longer contributes to the strength or the integrity of the cornea. The thin layer of corneal tissue removed by the laser to correct your vision is also no longer part of the cornea's strength. The corneal tissue remaining after the creation of the corneal flap and the ablation must be thick enough for cornea health. The general rule of thumb is that at least 250μ (some say 300) must remain for eye health. If the remaining cornea is too thin, it may gradually thin out over time (ectasia), leaving you more nearsighted than before you started. Corneal thickness varies from individual to individual and must always be measured before LVC.

Let's consider whether or not a −8.00 D myopic patient would be a good LASIK candidate. To correct every diopter of myopia, approximately 12μ of corneal tissue must be removed. The most popular microkeratome, the Hansatome made by Bausch and Lomb, creates a corneal flap of either 160μ or 180μ. Simple math reveals that for our −8.00 D myope (8 x 12 = 96), 96μ must be ablated for vision to be fully corrected. If a 160μ flap is created, 256μ (160 + 96 = 256) of tissue will be removed from the structural integrity of the cornea.

If this patient has an initial corneal thickness of approximately 490μ, LASIK would leave behind only 234μ of corneal tissue. This violates the 250μ rule (490–160–96 = 234). The remaining cornea would not be strong enough following LASIK, making this patient a poor candidate. If the patient's cornea was 570μ thick, LASIK would be a good possibility (570-256 = 314μ), because it is safely over the 250μ residual requirement.

However, if the cornea is too thin for LASIK, the –8.00 myopic patient could still safely have PRK or LASEK. By avoiding a corneal flap, the only corneal tissue removed would be the 96μ of the ablation, leaving a healthy 394μ. The surface epithelium of the cornea regenerates completely, so in this example thickness is not an issue. If the cornea is abnormally thin, such as 440 microns, most ophthalmologists would not advise any LVC procedure at all.

Some patients with cornea surface abnormalities such as basement membrane dystrophy might be poor candidates for LASIK, but excellent candidates for Surface Ablation. Some medical conditions such as rheumatoid arthritis, ulcerative colitis, and other autoimmune diseases would make any LVC procedure inadvisable. Other issues, such as extremely large pupils or irregular corneas, can disqualify some patients from any LVC.

5

Are You a Good Candidate for Laser Vision Correction?

Determining Your Candidacy

Are you a candidate for LVC? Based on the previous chapters, you should have a good idea if LVC is for you, if freedom from glasses or contact lenses is enough motivation to have surgery. Deciding you want to have LVC does not mean you can have it—you must have suitable eyes and even a suitable personality to become a satisfied LVC patient. The typical LVC patient should be over age eighteen (many surgeons prefer over twenty-one), have a stable refraction for two years, be in good health, and be free of contraindications (discussed later in this chapter).

One of the most important factors that determines whether you can have LVC is your prescription. A high myopic, hyperopic, or astigmatic prescription may make LVC ill advised. Despite the broad guidelines recommended by each laser manufacturer (most laser companies are approved for treating myopes up to –14.00), every eye surgeon has a comfort level, beyond which the results from LVC would be too unpredictable to recommend to patients. Generally, myopes above –10.00 or –11.00 D and hyperopes above +5.00 or +6.00 D are less successful than those with lower levels of refractive error.

In myopia, the effect of LVC on your cornea is like flattening a mountain peak into a level plateau. If your cornea is flattened too much in an attempt to correct vision—let's say you're a –15.00 D myope—the quality of your vision will suffer, even if all your myopia is gone. Quality of vision is not well understood, but a cornea that is abnormally flat or steep may produce aberrations that adversely affect vision. A similar analogy exists for hyperopia, where converting a "plateau" cornea into a steep mountain may lead to inferior image quality. There are many exceptions to these guidelines, so each patient needs to discuss options with his or her physician. More on this later.

Whether you are nearsighted, farsighted or astigmatic, a candidate for laser vision surgery must have a refractive error that has been stable for a period of at least two years. As with most parts of our bodies, our eyes and vision change over the course of our lives. If you have been wearing glasses since childhood or teen years, you probably went through a period of time, generally through your mid-twenties, when your prescription changed almost yearly. After that point, even into your early thirties, there was probably little or no change in your refractive error, and it stabilized. This explains why vision correction surgery is not performed on teenagers, whose eyes may change even several times a year. A prescription that endures for a two-year period is a good indication that most of the change is over.

The second issue to address is your cornea, eye and general health. There are other conditions that may preclude individuals from becoming vision surgery candidates:

- Herpes infections of the cornea—any eye surgery, including LVC, may reactivate herpes of the cornea.

- Keratoconus—a corneal condition that results in a thin, irregular, steep cornea. In most cases, no LVC procedure is advisable since this may weaken the cornea even further over the lifetime of the patient. A customized wavefront surface treatment may be possible. Your eye doctor can best advise on this often complex area (see Chapter Nine).

- Excessive corneal scarring—scar tissue that affects corneal clarity would not be removed during LVC, so there would be no improvement in best corrected vision. An exception might be a superficial scar, which could be ablated during LVC.

• Cataracts may make LVC unnecessary because vision is corrected with the insertion of an intraocular lens implant during cataract surgery.

• Intraocular pressure in patients with glaucoma (high intraocular pressure) may be more difficult to measure accurately following LVC, so patients with glaucoma need to discuss this with their doctor.

• Certain autoimmune conditions including lupus, rheumatoid arthritis, and inflammatory bowel diseases may cause the cornea to become inflamed or weak, so LVC, which might further thin the cornea, may not be advisable. There are exceptions, so talk to your eye doctor.

• Pregnancy, lactation, or menopause may cause unpredictable corneal healing.

• Severely dry eyes—LASIK, and to a much lesser degree Surface Ablation, may cause dryness of the cornea, and a dry cornea will not provide the same crisp vision as a moist, smooth cornea. A severely dry eye may weaken vision. Most dryness, however, can be treated, and some form of LVC is possible in most cases.

• Certain drugs such as Imitrex for migraine, Accutane for acne, and Cordarone for heart problems may affect your candidacy for surgery by causing irregular healing of the cornea.

The contraindications above are not absolute. A thorough understanding of your specific vision condition, accompanied by a discussion of all your options with your eye doctor, should enable you to decide whether LVC is still appropriate for you.

Surface Ablation Option

Your ophthamologist may recommend Surface Ablation instead of LASIK if you have one or more of the following conditions:

- Thin corneas

- Extremely flat or extremely steep corneas, both of which increase the likelihood of LASIK flap problems

- Extremely dry eyes, which can be aggravated by LASIK

- Extremely deep set eyes or very tight, slit-like lids, which can prevent the microkeratome from creating a good flap

- Loose epithelium (basement membrane dystrophy)

- Aberrations and other imperfections of the corneal surface

Avoiding a flap complication is not possible in all LASIK patients. A LASIK operation perfectly performed by the most experienced and skilled surgeon can still result in an incomplete, thin, or irregular flap, leading to healing problems such as striae, folds, or even a slipped flap. The use of the IntraLase laser to create the flap has reduced but not eliminated flap problems. If your eye doctor feels that you are in one of the higher risk categories, it may be best to avoid LASIK and choose Surface Ablation instead. The actual laser treatment to correct your vision in both LASIK and Surface Ablation is the same. More importantly, the results are the same, so the extra healing time may well be worth the extra safety of Surface Ablation. Approximately 5% of patients fare better with Surface Ablation, while 95% are good candidates for LASIK.

It's Up to You

Thanks to science and technology, your ophthalmologist now has the tools necessary to perform a thorough and comprehensive exam of your entire eye and cornea. Keratometry and pachymetry measure the curvature and thickness of your cornea, and the corneal topographer generates a detailed topographical map of its surface. The more advanced aberrometer reveals a diagnostic portrait of the imperfections and aberrations of your entire optical system. Once the data is reviewed, your ophthalmologist can discuss the suitability of your eyes for the operation. Just as Marcy Syms believes the educated consumer is her best customer, the educated patient, one who understands the procedure—what is done and why it works—and is fully cognizant of the potential for problems or complications, is the best patient. To become an educated patient is the reason you are reading this book!

Having eyes suitable for LVC is only half the equation for a satisfied patient. The other half of the equation must be a realistic mind-set with regards to expectations and motivation.

If you expect perfect vision with LVC, with a guarantee of a life totally free of glasses or contact lenses, then LVC is not for you. Any patient who is considering LVC must be prepared to wear glasses part-time. Part-time may mean while driving at night, sitting in the bleachers at Yankee Stadium, or reading fine print, but anticipating the need to wear glasses occasionally is a realistic expectation. Not all LVC patients must wear glasses part-time (most do not), but planning for the possibility will prevent disappointment.

Refraction, eye health, and corneal integrity are all factors used to determine whether vision surgery is an option for you, but a realistic expectation is an equally important factor. Wearing a pair of glasses only when driving at night or looking at a newspaper is a dramatic improvement over having to put glasses on every morning in order to see the alarm clock. Knowing this prior to surgery is the key to success.

6

LVC Operation Day

The preparation for LASIK and Surface Ablation is similar. Surgery is performed using anesthetic eye drops, is usually painless, and generally takes just a few minutes per eye. Having surgery on both eyes in the same day is more common with LASIK than with Surface Ablation, because the more rapid vision recovery of LASIK permits most LASIK patients to function normally the next day. Surface Ablation is often done on each eye a week apart, since vision can take that long to recover. Having PRK or epi-LASIK on both eyes at the same time may leave you too blurred to work for a few days, but some patients still prefer bilateral same-day surgery just to get everything done at one time. You and your eye doctor will have decided on separate or same day surgery ahead of time. It is a good idea to have a friend or relative accompany you home, especially if both eyes are done together.

LVC is usually performed in your eye doctor's office or in an open access laser center—an office where the laser is used by several eye doctors on the staff. A mild sedative, such as oral Valium, is often helpful to calm any last minute jitters and to make you more relaxed and comfortable during the procedure. Antibiotic drops are often started a few days prior to the procedure and continued for a few days after surgery. Contact lens wearers will have stopped wearing contact lenses for 1-2 weeks or up to a month or more—less for soft and more for gas permeable lenses. Contact lenses can alter the shape of the cornea, which, in turn, can alter your true refraction and reduce your chances for a successful outcome. Women should thoroughly remove all eye makeup several days before LVC. Perfume or cologne should not be worn on surgery day because fumes have the potential to alter the laser beam. Air quality, temperature, and humidity are tightly controlled in the room containing the laser.

A specially trained ophthalmic laser technician will operate the laser, and a second technician may assist the doctor. The untreated eye will be covered with an eye shield so only the eye receiving surgery can focus on the fixation light in the laser microscope without interference from the other eye. The operating microscope attached to the laser delivery console will give your ophthalmologist a clear, magnified view of your cornea throughout the procedure.

After several anesthetic eye drops are administered, an adhesive drape—usually made from clear surgical plastic—is taped over your eyelashes to prevent lashes or debris from falling on the surgical field and potentially causing an infection. An eyelid speculum—a spring-like clamp—is painlessly positioned between your lids to keep your eyes open wide. You will be required to look at the fixation light in the microscope, relax, and keep your eyes open. Your cooperation will help ensure a smooth procedure. Remember, there is virtually no pain during any type of LVC.

After your eyelids are cleaned, the eyelashes draped, and the speculum inserted between your lids, one or more alignment marks are made on your cornea with a blue, washable marking pen. These marks overlap the flap edge, so when the flap is repositioned and smoothed down at the end of the treatment, the marks line up, ensuring that the flap is repositioned correctly. The alignment marks, mostly used in LASIK, are washed away by your tears in a few hours.

The LASIK procedure starts with the creation of the corneal flap by the automated microkeratome. Most microkeratomes consist of two parts—a suction ring that resembles a metal washer attached to a vacuum tube, and the microkeratome head that creates the flap and acts like a carpenter's plane. In addition to raising the pressure inside your eye and making the cornea firm enough for the flap to be cut, the suction ring holds your eye perfectly still during the procedure and acts as a platform and track for the microkeratome. Once the proper suction is achieved, your doctor will use a small, plastic, cone-shaped instrument called a handheld tonometer to quickly ascertain that the intraocular pressure is sufficiently high to perform the operation. Flap problems, such as an incomplete flap, irregular flap, or a thin flap can occur if the pressure in the eye is not high enough. The increased pressure will cause your vision to darken for about fifteen seconds. Your doctor will ask if your vision is dark as a way to confirm the increased pressure before stepping on the microkeratome foot pedal to make the flap. There is no pain, only a sensation of pressure. When the flap is made with the IntraLase, there is less sensation of pressure and less chance of a flap problem. Once the flap is created, your eye is ready for laser treatment.

Depending on your eyeglass prescription and whether you are near-sighted or farsighted, the laser ablation can last anywhere from five to ten seconds to over a minute or two. As you continue to look at the fixation light, you will hear a clicking sound as the laser emits painless pulses of the cool laser light. Most excimer lasers have a tracker, so if your eye does stray slightly, the laser beam will stay centered on your cornea as it tracks your involuntary eye movement. A laser treatment that is not sufficiently centered can result in reduced BCVA, glare, halos, and distortion, so the tracker is an important improvement in LVC surgery. If your eye moves too much, the laser will automatically stop until you regain fixation on the target in the microscope. If you are having a custom ablation treatment (VISX Wavescan) the laser will also lock on to the architecture of your iris, further ensuring a centered treatment. The centration of the laser beam is calibrated each morning and its accuracy checked throughout the day. Throughout the treatment, your eye doctor will be monitoring your eye through the microscope.

Once the ablation is completed, your eye doctor will precisely reposition the flap, using the alignment marks as a guide. He will have first gently irrigated beneath the flap, using a mild saline solution to remove any debris left by your tears, eyelids, or microkeratome. The flap is given a final smoothing with a miniature sponge that resembles a tiny paintbrush, and then allowed to dry for several minutes before the speculum between your eyelids is removed. The procedure is now complete.

If you are having surgery on both eyes, the newly treated eye is patched and the procedure is repeated on your other eye.

You'll be escorted to a dimly lit recovery room to relax, and your companion may rejoin you there. Most surgeons prefer that you keep your eyes closed in the recovery area so the flap can begin to stabilize and rebond to your cornea.

Each surgeon has his or her own protocol for surgery and the recovery period, which includes not rubbing your eyes and careful showering. I encourage my patients to keep their eyes closed or take a nap for an hour upon arriving at home in order to give the flap a chance to start healing. Most surgeons will provide their patients with a goody bag containing a plastic shield and tape to protect your eye during sleep (a good idea for at least the first night) and antibiotic and anti-inflammatory drops.

The average patient is able to resume regular activities and return to work within twenty-four hours of the procedure. Avoid rubbing your eye for at least a week to prevent dislodging the flap. For a week or two following the operation, you should wear a headband at the gym to prevent sweat from entering your eyes. Avoid hot tubs and swimming pools because they are possible sources of contamination. Sports that may result in an eye injury, such as tennis and basketball, should also be avoided for a week or two. Noncontact sports, such as golf, cycling, or jogging can be enjoyed sooner.

Your eyesight will remain blurry for several hours immediately following the procedure, but a night's sleep will usually improve vision dramatically. Though each patient is different and eye healing rate varies, even within the same patient, by the next day most patients will already be able to pass a vision test for driving—20/40 uncorrected vision.

PRK, Epi-LASIK, and LASEK

From the patient's perspective, there is little difference between having LASIK and Surface Ablation because the laser ablation is the same in all three forms of LVC. The main difference for the patient is more discomfort after surgery and longer healing, both helped by oral medication, eye drops, and the bandage soft contact lens used at the conclusion of Surface Ablation. This contact lens is placed on your eye by the doctor or technician and acts as a bandage to cover your cornea while it heals. Surface Ablation, unlike LASIK, requires longer than twenty-four hours for vision to improve to the point where you can drive. In the end, the results are the same—welcome to a world without eyeglasses or contact lenses.

7

Understanding Risks and Complications

For the vast majority of the greater than one million patients undergoing LVC each year, the results will be everything anticipated—an uneventful procedure, rapid, predictable healing, and eyesight so good that glasses or contacts will be a thing of the past. For a small group of LVC patients, anywhere from 1%–5% of the total, the results may be slightly disappointing. Healing may take longer than expected, vision may not be as sharp as anticipated, and an enhancement or other surgical procedure may be necessary to fine-tune the results. Unforeseen side effects may occur. You should understand what side effects can occur, what can go wrong, and what the chances are of having a less than perfect result.

As we shall see, complications vary greatly and do not necessarily adversely affect the final outcome of LVC. For example, during LASIK, the surface epithelial layer of the cornea may loosen (epithelial slide) or partly fall off (abrasion) when the flap is made by the microkeratome. Although healing will be slower than if this complication had not occurred, the outcome is usually excellent. True complications—those events that can blur, distort, or cloud your vision and cannot be fixed by glasses or contact lenses are very rare, about one in ten thousand. Infection, which can leave your eye permanently cloudy and require a corneal transplant, is extremely rare, perhaps one in ten to twenty thousand. Your eye doctor will prescribe antibiotic drops before the procedure that will further reduce the risk of infection.

The following list explains the most common LVC complications. The list is not complete, and some complications are so rare as almost never to occur, such as a patient dying from a fatal heart attack during LVC. I know of no such occurrence, but it is possible, as in, "anything is possible." But even the most common complications are unlikely to occur in the average patient. Complications that cause loss of best corrected visual acuity (BCVA) are more serious than other complications. Doctors worry less about complications that are correctable with glasses or contact lenses than about those complications that leave the patient with permanent, uncorrectable loss of vision, however mild. If a patient is expecting 20/20 after LVC, disappointment may occur if uncorrected vision is less than this. But if glasses or contacts can correct vision back to 20/20, there has not been a loss of that all important BCVA. In almost all instances, the eye will remain as healthy as before LVC, and glasses will likely be needed only part-time at most, or not at all.

Under-and Overcorrections

Undercorrections and overcorrections are not really complications, because an LVC procedure can be technically perfect but your cornea may respond more (overcorrection) or less (undercorrection) than in other patients. An under-or overcorrection results in retention of some degree of a myopic, hyperopic, or astigmatic refractive error following surgery. An undercorrection may not noticeably affect your vision and may only appear when you look at the eye chart during a follow-up exam. In some cases—such as nearsighted patients over forty—an undercorrection may be desirable, delaying for several years or more the need for reading glasses. Undercorrections are more likely in patients with higher levels of myopia, hyperopia, or astigmatism.

The significance of an over-or undercorrection depends upon many factors, including your initial refraction and your age. If a –8.00 D myope has LVC and is undercorrected by only half or three-quarters of a diopter, it means that almost 95% of the –8.00 D refractive error was corrected, and the undercorrection may be of little or no consequence. On the other hand, if a −1.50 D myope retains the same −0.50 or −0.75 D undercorrection, only 50% of the refractive error would have been corrected—an unacceptable result for both patient and doctor.

In these two examples, an overcorrection would result in a refractive error of +0.50 D or a +0.75 D. Whether or not retaining +0.50 D or +0.75 D would have a significant effect on vision depends more on the patient's age than on the original refractive error.

For a twenty-five-year-old patient, the extra focusing required to correct the small amount of induced hyperopia would be effortless and automatic because more than enough reserve focusing power remains in the eye of a twenty-five-year-old. In fact, the same patient would be unaware of the overcorrection, would have 20/20 uncorrected vision, and would be quite satisfied. A forty-five-year-old patient, whether originally a −8.00 D or −1.50 D and ending up overcorrected to a refractive error of +0.50 D or +0.75 D, would be less happy compared to the twenty-five-year-old patient. At forty-five, the reserve focusing power is very low, and reading glasses would be required to correct the sudden burden of overcorrection and hyperopia. It is often more desirable to err on the side of an undercorrection in a forty-five-year-old to avoid overcorrecting.

In monovision, one eye of a myopic patient is intentionally left slightly nearsighted in order to give some reading vision for items such as a menu or price tag and to avoid reliance on reading glasses. Similarly, a +2.00 D forty-five-year-old hyperope might aim for an overcorrection to −1.00 D in one eye, so reading glasses would not be necessary except for small print. A +4.00 D hyperope would probably not be able to have monovision, because LVC is not as reliable over +4.00 D, and the treatment programmed into the laser would have to be at least +5.00 D for the +4.00 D patient to end up −1.00 D. The subtle nuances of over-and undercorrection should be discussed with your doctor. The higher your prescription, the higher the chances of over-and undercorrection but in the average patient the chances are usually less than 5%.

If you are unhappy with over- or undercorrected vision, you will need a second procedure known as an enhancement. Myopes with a slightly thin cornea may not have enough residual thickness for an enhancement following an initial LASIK operation. Enhancement procedures almost always follow the same pattern as the initial LASIK. Rather than cutting a new flap, the surgeon breaks the seal of the original flap and lifts it up and out of the way for the new laser treatment. Once this additional laser ablation is completed, the flap is replaced as in the original treatment. Occasionally, PRK or LASEK is performed as an enhancement for LASIK. If your original procedure was PRK or LASEK, the same procedure will usually be used for the enhancement operation, although LASIK can often be done instead. Enhancements carry the same low risk of infection as the original procedure, but the risk of epithelial ingrowth is higher.

Regression

Regression is the tendency for the eye to drift back toward its original refractive error—a delayed undercorrection. In most cases, this drifting back is minimal, and you need not worry that you will suddenly find yourself back at your original refractive error. Regression can occur as early as one or two months after the original surgery or more than a year later. The higher your refractive error, the greater is the chance for regression. That is why a –6.00 D myope with immediate post-surgery results of +0.50 D, will probably suffer a slight regression of 0.50 diopters and will finish happily with a zero refractive error. If the regression is significant, an enhancement procedure can be performed.

Glare Disability—Starbursts and Halos

Glare disability refers to a problem with light at night, such as seeing starbursts and halos while driving or looking at any light source in the dark. Glare disability can be a serious problem after LVC, making a patient with perfect 20/20 vision unhappy. The cause of halos and starbursts is somewhat controversial and was initially thought to be due to large pupils in the dark, such as at night. However, many patients with large pupils have no glare problems, and some with small pupils do. The cause may be in the centration of the laser treatment over the pupil, and the smoothness of the laser treatment itself. Glare disability, starbursts, and halos are much less common now, because surgeons more carefully measure pupil size before surgery and use smoother, wider laser treatment zones. For example, if the pupil dilates to 8 mm in the dark and the laser treatment or ablation is 6 mm, light from headlights and streetlights will hit the edge of the lasered/unaltered cornea and be diffracted into starbursts or halos. In daylight or in a lighted room, the pupil will usually be smaller than the 6 mm ablation zone, so glare disability is not an issue.

Besides correcting your vision, most laser treatments now smooth out the transition zone between the lasered and unlasered part of your cornea. This minimizes any glare that may occur if your pupil dilates too much at night. In general, glare is more of an issue with myopes, and the higher your prescription, the more likely it is that you may have some glare.

For patients with large pupils, custom ablation may be advisable because glare is less likely with a custom laser treatment (Chapter Nine). Ophthalmologists debate the relationship between glare and pupil size, but it is still a good idea to be aware of this issue before you decide to have LVC.

Other factors can also cause glare. Rarely, the cornea heals abnormally, causing the surface of the cornea to be irregular. If the eye drifts off-center during the procedure and if the ablation is not sufficiently centered on the cornea (decentered ablation), glare or poor vision may result. However, precise eye trackers on the laser make a decentered ablation much less common now.

Whatever the cause, glare disability in the form of starbursts and other annoying reflections often disappear in three to six months after LVC. If symptoms persist, new approaches using WaveScan-driven laser treatments promise to help these patients.

Central Island

Central Island, now rare, is another potential LVC complication that results in ghost images and other visual disturbances postoperatively. These visual aberrations occur because a small area in the center of the treatment zone received fewer laser pulses than the surrounding tissue. This may be caused by a plume of lasered tissue that rises up from the center of the laser zone to partially block the remaining laser pulses from passing through to the center of the cornea. Diagnosis of central island is made with the corneal topographer, which produces a digitized map of the corneal surface and will identify any raised islands within the treatment zone. Central islands often will disappear within a few months, but in other cases, an additional smoothing laser treatment may be needed. Newer excimer laser systems now have anticentral island software that produces additional laser pulses as part of the initial treatment to prevent this complication.

Flap Complications

Complications involving the corneal flap are confined to LASIK because there is no flap in Surface Ablation. Corneal flap complications can be completely eliminated by choosing Surface Ablation, so why do the majority of eye surgeons and their patients still choose LASIK? Most do so because LASIK heals faster and the chances of a flap complication are unlikely, especially when the flap is made with the IntraLase laser, rather than a mechanical microkeratome. Although flap complications can occur even in the most skilled surgical hands, they generally occur in less than 1% of patients. They include the following:

• Poor, partial, or incomplete flap—When the flap is created by an automated instrument, mechanical failure of the microkeratome during the fifteen to twenty seconds it takes to create the flap can result in a partial or incomplete flap. Usually this failure will not affect vision and the surgery can be repeated in several months, giving the incompletely cut flap an opportunity to heal before a new flap is made. Sometimes, a thin line of scar tissue can remain in the center of the cornea in the visual axis causing reduced acuity or distortion. Rarely, a corneal transplant will be needed. A poor flap, one that is too thick, too thin, or irregular, occurs in about one out of every four hundred to five hundred patients. If the flap is imperfect, the laser ablation should be aborted. The flap is replaced and a new procedure is performed several months later. A poor flap is usually due to some loss of suction by the microkeratome during the creation of the flap. Loss of suction may be caused by a microkeratome mechanical problem, such as the keratome hitting the eyelid speculum, very tight eyelids that are being squeezed shut during the procedure, or the keratome jamming in its track on the suction ring. Patient cooperation, aided by sedation if necessary, is important for a successful outcome. Microkeratomes are amazingly accurate and extremely dependable. The surgeon inspects and tests the device before every procedure, and the blade that makes the incision is discarded after each patient. The chance of a mechanical failure or other mishap causing a bad corneal flap or an uneven incision is highly unlikely. The IntraLase laser is extremely reliable, but not infallible, and a poor flap can rarely occur when the flap is made with a femtosecond laser rather than a blade.

• Epithelial erosion—The surface of the cornea is covered by a plastic wrap-like sheet of cells called the epithelium. It covers the cornea in much the same way as skin covers your body. Although the attachment of the epithelium to the underlying corneal stroma is usually strong, in some patients (more in women than men, and more often in women over forty), the attachment contains weak spots. The result is that when the keratome passes back and forth to make the flap, some epithelial tissue may be rubbed off, resulting in a corneal erosion. Usually the final success of LASIK is unaffected, but to aid in healing a bandage soft contact lens is placed on the cornea and left in place until the abrasion heals, usually in a day or two. Certain corneal abnormalities, such as basement membrane dystrophy, can help identify patients who are at risk for epithelial erosions during standard LASIK with the microkeratome. These patients may be more suitable for Surface Ablation or LASIK using the IntraLase to make the flap. Frustration for both patient and doctor occurs when a cornea that appears healthy suffers an erosion, despite the lack of any indication that it might occur. If an erosion does occur, there is an increased risk of inflammation (DLK, see below) and other flap problems during healing, but the results are usually excellent once healing is complete. If you suffer a large erosion or if the entire epithelium is loose (epithelial slide), your eye doctor will probably postpone treating your second eye until your first eye has completely healed. With a small epithelial defect, surgery on the second eye can usually proceed.

- Flap folds, wrinkles, striae—A LASIK procedure that proceeds smoothly (more than 99% do), should result in a cornea that is as clear and as smooth as the cornea was in its presurgery state. In some patients, the flap may heal with fine wrinkles, or stria, occasionally reducing vision. If this happens, you may need a second procedure to smooth or stretch the striae. Striae that are treated within the first few days or week after LASIK are easier to eliminate than those that are treated weeks or months later, but persistent striae can still be eliminated even years after the procedure. Striae occur for several reasons, primarily due to a mismatch between the shape of the flap and the newly lasered, underlying stroma. This mismatch is more likely to occur in highly myopic patients, when there is greater flattening of the cornea to correct vision. If the flap, which may try to retain its curvature, does not conform to the newly flattened corneal stroma, wrinkles or stria can result, interfering with vision.

- Another cause of wrinkles or striae is flap slippage. Before the flap is made, the surgeon places one or more marks on the cornea with a blue or purple surgical marking pen. The marks straddle the seam of the flap, so that when the flap is replaced after laser ablation, the marks should line up, ensuring that the flap fits exactly where it was before the mircrokeratome cut the flap. If the flap slips or moves out of position, either because the patient inadvertently rubs the eye or forcefully blinks or squeezes the eye shut, wrinkles or striae could develop. Not all striae need to be repaired, and not all striae affect vision. Sometimes very delicate, fine striae form just under the surface of the cornea because of its new shape. These micro striae usually do not affect vision and do not require treatment. Larger, visually significant or macro striae need prompt attention before they become permanent. Treatment of striae and slipped flaps depends on severity and duration and varies from simply relifting and replacing, to suturing the flap in place for several weeks. Deciding which patients with microstriae need treatment and which do not is often an art more than a science. It is based as much on the patient's symptoms, such as loss of best corrected vision, as on the judgement of the doctor. Some doctors treat virtually no microstria, allowing the surface epithelium to grow in and around the microstria, evening out the surface. Some doctors will lift, stretch and smooth out the cornea to eliminate even the slightest amount of microstria. If you do have microstria, as opposed to macrostria which need immediate treatment, your doctor will discuss your options.

Flap-related Complications

Certain complications can occur in the presence of a LASIK flap but are not in the flap itself:

- Sands of the Sahara or diffuse lamellar keratitis (DLK)—As with any surgery or injury to the human body (and the eye is no exception), a certain amount of white blood cell inflammations is normal. About 1% of patients experience a temporary inflammatory reaction called diffuse lamellar keratitis or DLK, beneath the flap. In DLK, an excessive amount of white blood cells accumulates in the protected space under the flap (lamellar). These cells form layers that resemble miniature sand dunes. The exact cause is unknown, but is likely due to a combination of factors including over-response by the body's immune system. DLK, generally beginning during the first or second day after surgery, can occur after even the most expertly performed LASIK. Patients with DLK may not have any symptoms at all or may experience a degree of blurred vision and tearing that can worsen over several days to several weeks. Treatment includes frequent use of anti-inflammatory drops, oral steroids (cortisone), or under-flap irrigation to remove inflammation. Prompt treatment usually completely restores vision. If left untreated, scarring and serious flap damage can occur.

- Epithelial ingrowth—In LASIK, the U-shaped flap disrupts the surface epithelial layer and when the flap is smoothed down after the laser ablation, new epithelial cells grow across the thin "gutter," or seam. Rarely, these cells can grow under the flap, a condition called epithelial ingrowth. In most cases, the epithelial cells stop growing on their own and slowly dissolve or disappear. In some cases, the epithelial cells continue to grow, forming a sheet of tissue under the edge of the flap and across the center of the cornea, the critically important "visual axis." This sheet of cells can compromise flap health and severely reduce vision. Treatment includes lifting the flap and removing all traces of epithelial cells. Even with meticulous removal, however, it is not uncommon for microscopic nests of cells to remain, resulting in reoccurrence of the epithelial ingrowth. Suturing down the flap usually stops the ingrowth, and sutures are removed within a few weeks. Epithelial ingrowth is more common after epithelial erosion or abrasion during LASIK, or if the flap is relifted to treat striae or for an enhancement.

- Dry eyes—Tears are critical for healthy eyes. Without tears, your cornea would be dry and lose clarity. Two systems in the eye produce tears. The tears that come from crying, peeling onions or laughing to the point of tears come from the lacrimal gland, situated just underneath the outer portion of the upper lid. These tears are minimally affected by LASIK.

The other tear-producing system consists of thousands of microscopic tear glands embedded in the thin mucous membrane that lines the inside of the upper and lower eyelids. These glands produce tears continuously and are affected by LASIK, although in the vast majority of people, only temporarily. Why only the eyelid system is affected is not completely clear but may be due partly to the corneal nerves that are severed when the flap is made. These nerves are involved in maintaining cornea moisture. When cut, they can no longer function until they regenerate, usually about three months later. In the "hinge," the area of the flap that is not cut, the corneal nerves are intact and will continue to function to keep tears flowing and provide the cornea with limited moisture. The use of artificial tears and "punctum plugs" to prevent tears from draining away are both treatments for dry eye and will usually control symptoms until the eye's own natural tear production returns. In rare cases, dry eye may be permanent and debilitating, a potential complication best discovered in the preoperative exam and evaluation. If dry eye is likely to be a problem, Surface Ablation, rather than LASIK, may be the best choice because corneal nerves are cut only in LASIK.

• Debris under the flap—A small amount of debris can accumulate under the flap. The debris can result from normal eyelid oil and flakes, from material on the surgical instruments, even from lint or other foreign material in the air. As a routine step during the surgery, the surgeon will irrigate under the flap with a sterile solution of water and electrolytes, just after the laser ablation and just before the flap is repositioned. Despite the irrigation, some debris can remain. It usually has no effect on vision or the success of the procedure.

• Corneal ectasia—Ectasia is a medical term for thinning, such as the cornea thinning after LASIK. Although the LASIK corneal flap adheres to the corneal bed after it is smoothed down and contributes to focusing and corneal clarity as it did before the flap was made, it no longer contributes to the structural integrity and strength of the cornea. That is why your surgeon calculates how much corneal tissue will remain after subtracting the thickness of the corneal flap and the thickness of the tissue removed by the laser. Most surgeons use 250μ as the benchmark number required for cornea health. Although the label on the microkeratome may indicate the flap thickness will be 160μ, and the ultrasonic pachymeter might read the corneal thickness before surgery as 520μ, slight inaccuracies are possible, leaving the cornea thinner than planned. For some patients, even 250μ may not be sufficient corneal thickness for long-term stability of the cornea. This reduced stability can lead to a bulging or steepening of the cornea, resulting in a return of myopia or in deformity or distortion of the cornea, requiring, in rare instances, a corneal transplant. Careful preoperative planning should enable your eye doctor to avoid ectasia, but in very rare instances, it can happen despite your surgeon's best efforts. Surface Ablation may be a good option if you have borderline corneal thickness.

Infection

The occurrence of infection of the cornea after LVC is very low. Most eye surgeons will prescribe antibiotic drops for several days prior to the procedure and instill antibiotic drops at the conclusion of the surgery. Most doctors also advise their patients to continue using the antibiotic drops for several days after the operation. A corneal infection, much more serious than conjunctivitis (pink eye), can potentially lead to scarring of the cornea and reduced vision. Infections following LVC may be caused by unusual and resistant bacteria, rather than more readily treatable bacteria such as staphylococcus or streptococcus. If the infection occurs under the LASIK flap, antibiotic drops may have trouble penetrating the flap, resulting in a less than optimal concentration of antibiotic needed to fight the infection. In some cases, the flap may need to be lifted or removed to successfully treat an infection. With Surface Ablation, infections are more easily treated, but resistant organisms can still pose a problem.

Fortunately, infection after LVC is rare, even though it is a less sterile procedure than intraocular surgery (surgery on the inside of the eye) such as cataract or glaucoma surgery. Intraocular surgery occurs in an operating room, where doctors and nurses wear sterile gowns and gloves. The operating microscope is adorned with sterile handles for adjusting and focusing, and the patient is prepped using an iodine scrub on the eyelids and part of the face.

In LVC, the instruments are as sterile as in any other eye surgery, and the eyelids are often cleansed with antiseptic. But since there is no surgery on the inside of the eye—where even the slightest infection in the "closed system" of the eyes can be devastating—the rigorous sterile technique is less intense. Nonetheless, the LVC surgeon and staff do whatever is necessary, such as frequent applications of antibiotic drops, to minimize any chance of infection.

Corneal Haze

Corneal haze is a complication unique to Surface Ablation. As the new epithelium regenerates to cover the cornea's surface, a grayish substance can accumulate in between the epithelial cells. This substance, technically called collagen matrix, can reduce vision despite a perfectly performed operation. The more myopic the patient, the more this substance accumulates after healing occurs, and the greater the chance of haze.

Typically haze does not appear until months after surgery. Mild degrees of haze may not affect vision, while severe haze can reduce vision dramatically. Fortunately, haze usually disappears slowly over time, and vision returns. If haze does not fade, it can be surgically removed. Haze is less common with the latest generation of lasers that ablate with a smoother profile. It is also less common in myopic prescriptions less than 6 diopters. Epi-LASIK and LASEK may create less haze than PRK, but a definitive study on this issue has been inconclusive. Haze is rare in surface ablation for hyperopia or astigmatism.

8

How to Find the Right Eye Doctor

If you need an eye exam, or you are interested in LVC, you may find yourself in the office of either an ophthalmologist or an optometrist. What is the difference, and who will do your eye surgery? An ophthalmologist is a physician (or M.D.—Doctor of Medicine), just as a cardiologist or neurosurgeon is also a physician. An ophthalmologist has attended undergraduate school, four years of medical school, and one year of internship—rotating through various medical specialties and subspecialties. To specialize in ophthalmology, a physician must complete a three-or four-year residency in ophthalmology, where in-depth studies include ocular anatomy, physiology, pathology, diseases, and surgery. Some ophthalmologists take extra training in a fellowship to specialize in one area or disease of the eye such as glaucoma, the retina, or the cornea.

Optometrists also attend undergraduate school, followed by four years of optometry school, where they study the eye in courses similar to those in an ophthalmology residency, including the diagnosis and treatment of eye disease. In addition, their schooling emphasizes the science of vision, refraction, and the fitting, formulation, and sale of eyeglasses and contact lenses. Although not physicians, and therefore not able to perform surgery, optometrists provide a valuable eye-care function. They perform eye examinations, diagnose eye disease, and in most states, prescribe topical eyedrops. Your optometrist can often tell if you are a good candidate for LVC or can refer you to an ophthalmologist.

So, how do you find a doctor competent to perform LVC? Although there is no foolproof method of finding the right ophthalmologist for your surgery, the following methods may be helpful.

Staying with Your Current Ophthalmologist

If you are already under the care of a board-certified ophthalmologist who performs LVC (not all do), trust his or her skills, and are satisfied with the eye care you have received over the years, you probably need to look no further. Most eye surgeons are board certified, indicating that they have demonstrated an in-depth knowledge by passing a rigorous examination administered by the American Board of Ophthalmology.

If you do need to start with a new ophthalmologist, I recommend that you seek one with experience performing LVC. Although even the most experienced LVC surgeon started with a first patient, experience is a factor in successful LVC. How do you measure experience? Are twenty-five operations enough to pronounce your eye doctor experienced? There is no magic number, but most ophthalmologists would agree that an ophthalmologist would need to perform at least twenty-five to fifty LVC procedures to feel comfortable, and one hundred to two hundred to be even more competent. As in all professions, skill levels vary. An experienced eye surgeon who has done thousands of other eye operations, such as cataract or glaucoma surgery, may need to have performed fewer LVC procedures than a less-experienced surgeon to be considered competent. All ophthalmologists who perform LVC must attend training and educational courses given by different excimer laser companies and be certified by the company whose laser he or she will be using. In addition, most microkeratome companies provide similar courses and require similar certification.

In addition to verifying the certification and LVC experience level of the surgeon you are considering, it's important to ask the eye doctor about his complication and enhancement rates. Both should be low, approaching no more than 1% or 2%. Knowing your surgeon's outcome statistics would also be helpful. What percentage of patients achieves at least 20/40, what percentage achieves 20/20? What percentage has a loss of BCVA?

Board certification and experience are not substitutes for one of the most important skills a physician can possess—good judgment. Good judgment is the ability to instinctively know which patients have realistic expectations and which ones do not. Good judgment is knowing which corneas need treatment for microstria and which ones only require observation. Good judgment and excellent surgical skills are important qualities of a competent and qualified eye surgeon. If your ophthalmologist meets the above criteria, then there is no need to consider anyone else.

Referral from Your Optometrist

If your regular eye doctor is an optometrist, you might want to ask for a recommendation for an ophthalmologist who performs LVC. Who is better than an eye-care professional for recommending a good eye surgeon? This approach usually works well, provided your optometrist has your best interests at heart. However, some optometrists comanage their LVC patients with an ophthalmologist and receive a comanagement fee for their work. This arrangement might not influence your optometrist's referral to an ophthalmologist, but as a patient, you should be aware of this practice. Comanagement works like this: An optometrist refers the patient to an ophthalmologist for LVC. The ophthalmologist completes all necessary testing, including deciding whether the patient is a good candidate for LVC and reviewing informed consent, risks, and complications. After surgery, the ophthalmologist will see the patient for one or two postoperative visits, after which all other follow-up care will be assumed by the referring optometrist. The surgical fee often includes the comanagement fee and is paid to the optometrist by the ophthalmologist. Comanaging LVC patients arose in rural areas where there were fewer eye surgeons than optometrists. Comanagement works well, as long as financial reward does not affect referrals and quality eye care.

Referral from a Family Doctor

A referral from your family doctor is a good way to find an ophthalmologist for an eye exam and treatment of common eye problems such as glaucoma, cataracts, and pink eye. LVC is specialized and general practitioners may not know enough about the skills of eye doctor colleagues to make a reliable recommendation. A phone call from your family doctor to one or two ophthalmologists to whom he or she refers patients would help you find an eye doctor who is competent to perform LVC. If you trust your family doctor, you should trust his referrals, too. If none of his colleagues perform LVC, they would be able to recommend someone who does.

Lay Recommendations

A recommendation from a friend, relative, or coworker who has had successful LVC may seem like a good way to find the right LVC surgeon, but it does not guarantee similar success for you. Was your friend as nearsighted or as far sighted as you? Did you both have the same expectations? LVC in the hands of a well-trained ophthalmologist has a low complication rate, and it is likely that your surgery will go as well as that of your friend or coworker, but his success does not guarantee yours.

Recommendations from Advertising

Physicians are held to higher standards than those of other professionals, and catchy advertisements and self-promotion seem less appropriate in medicine than in other professions. Although doctors who advertise may be as skilled and as caring as purported in the ads, relying solely on ads is not a good way to find the best doctor for your eye surgery. Ads cost money—payment for the ads should not be a factor in your doctor's evaluation of your suitability for LVC. Ads may be a good starting point, or they may be one of several methods you use to find Dr. Right, but they should not be your only method.

Cost

Cost is a factor to consider in deciding whether to have LVC. Vision surgery, like cosmetic surgery, is elective surgery—it is at your discretion and not "medically necessary." But while refractive surgery and plastic surgery both enhance quality of life, most ophthalmologists do not consider refractive surgery to be cosmetic, since refractive surgery improves the function of the eye, not just the appearance. An example would be the –8.00 D myope who would be unable to see if he lost his glasses during an accident or a fire. One day after LVC he would be able to drive without glasses. Because LVC is elective, health insurance will rarely pay for all of it. But many plans, particularly those with a vision care component, will pay for a portion of the fee. With the growth of laser vision surgery, insurance plans that offer vision care and pay for glasses or contact lenses have found that paying at least part of the cost of LASIK can actually be cheaper than annually replacing contacts or glasses. Talk to your insurance plan administrators and your eye doctor as part of your LASIK decision-making process.

What can you expect to pay for the procedure? Expect to pay between $1500 and $3000 per eye, and in most cases, more for custom ablation. Enhancements for up to a year or more are often included in the fee. Price has become a confusing issue because marketing and advertising have proliferated. Advertising medical services has become part of the American commercial landscape, and, while it may have some positive aspects, such as increasing awareness of health care and consumer choice, presenting LVC as a commodity rather than surgery can give the patient a false sense of security. Though price should never be the primary factor in your decision, remember that low prices do not inevitably mean poor quality. In the recent past, corporate-owned, discount laser centers offered LASIK for $1,000 for both eyes. The surgery was usually of the highest caliber because good surgeons were hired to perform the same high-quality surgery that they offered to their own private patients. It was the high cost of advertising coupled with a low profit margin, rather than a quality issue, that drove most centers out of business.

Ask questions. Ask as many questions as you need to make a good decision. I hope this book helps you to know what to ask and to understand the answers you receive. Without knowledge of LVC, you won't know what you don't know. If you are not receiving adequate answers about what procedure will be best for your degree of refractive error and your vision needs, or if you feel that you are being pressured to get the procedure and eye health issues aren't the primary consideration, you should reevaluate your choice of an eye surgeon.

9

The Future

Wavefront Technology

LVC is the most revolutionary, rapidly changing area in ophthalmology. Refractive surgeons worldwide have vowed to reach the goal of super vision—"20/10 by 2010," and it may well become a reality in the near future. It is driven by innovations in LVC that will change the future of vision correction forever. One such innovation—wavefront technology—holds the most promise for "20/10 by 2010." First approved for clinical use in 2002, wavefront technology involves measuring the optical imperfections of the eye and then guiding the excimer laser to correct them. Used for many years to measure the quality of optical lenses in astronomy, wavefront technology is now available for use in LVC.

All human eyes suffer from optical aberrations or distortions. Low-order aberrations are the familiar sphere and cylinder of myopia, hyperopia, and astigmatism, measured through refraction and denoted by diopters on your prescription. Higher-order aberrations such as trefoil, coma, and other similarly unfamiliar terms cannot be measured with a standard refraction. Instead, they are measured with a complex, computerized instrument called an aberrometer. The aberrometer measures the total amount of aberrations in the eye, including the familiar refraction, and transforms this complex data into a wavefront map. To generate a wavefront map (called a WaveScan by VISX, the laser model I use), the aberrometer sends an infrared wave of light into the eye and analyzes the wave of light that is reflected. The more aberrations in the eye, usually in the cornea and lens, the more irregular the reflected wave of light will be. In a wavefront-guided LVC, aberrometer findings (the WaveScan), are transferred to a hard drive, and then loaded into the excimer laser. The laser ablation pattern to improve your vision is derived from the total set of aberrations in the WaveScan, including the refraction used in standard LVC.

To better understand wavefront technology, picture the surface of a pond, smooth and flat, undisturbed by wind. This is analogous to the ideal optical system, without any aberrations. If wind blows across the surface of the pond, or if a pebble is tossed into the water, the surface of the pond is disrupted by ripples. These surface ripples are aberrations. In general terms, the flatter and smoother your wavefront, the better your vision will be. Although no one has a perfectly flat wavefront, or a perfect optical system without aberration, most people have mainly second-order aberrations (myopia, hyperopia, and astigmatism), easily correctable by glasses or contact lenses. A wavefront-guided ablation that can correct the remaining third-order and higher aberration promises unsurpassed vision. As of this writing, four excimer laser systems have been approved by the Food and Drug Administration (FDA) for wavefront-guided laser treatments. Alcon Pharmaceutical's LADAR Wave Customized Ablation System received approval in October 2002, the VISX CustomVue System in May 2003, Bausch & Lomb's Zyoptix System in October 2003, and Allegretto's wavefront-guided WaveLight in August 2006. Results have been excellent, most patients having achieved 20/20 or better vision. Customized treatments are now approved for almost all levels of refractive errors, but as more studies are completed and more data becomes available, the range of approved treatments will be expanded.

Intralasik

Although the complication rate for LASIK is low, 1% or less, most complications are flap-related rather than laser-related. Flaps that are too thin, irregular, incomplete, contain a "button hole," or contain a large area of loose or abraded epithelium may give suboptimal results or may cause the surgeon to abort the laser step completely.

The precision of a flap created by a laser, rather than a micro-keratome with a steel blade, may greatly reduce or even eliminate serious flap problems. The IntraLase Corporation of Irvine, California, recently received FDA approval for just such a laser—the Femtosecond laser. The laser pulses, each lasting one quadrillionth of a second (femtosecond), are programmed to pass harmlessly through the surface of the cornea and create a flap of predetermined thickness. As with the standard mechanized microkeratome, a small hinge of tissue remains uncut, forming an area where the flap can be folded out of the way so that the excimer laser can reshape the cornea.

The entire IntraLase flap procedure takes less than thirty seconds, and with the use of standard anesthetic drops, is painless. There are several advantages to the IntraLase system. Flap thickness is more precise and predictable than with a microkeratome, where flap thickness can vary by 20µ to 30µ or more. Some patients with borderline cornea thickness may become eligible for IntraLase LASIK rather than PRK because the femtosecond laser can be programmed to make a thinner flap, leaving behind more residual corneal tissue.

With IntraLase, the likelihood of epithelial abrasion and incomplete flaps is greatly reduced, though not totally eliminated, because there is less friction on the cornea with IntraLase than with a microkeratome blade. Patients with surface cornea problems, such as basement membrane dystrophy, might become eligible for LASIK if the flap is made with a laser rather than a blade.

Another advantage of the IntraLase procedure is a more uniform flap thickness that may better fit into the cornea following laser ablation—like a manhole cover into the street. IntraLase does not eliminate other flap problems, such as stria and folds.

There are several potential disadvantages of using the Femtasecond laser to create the LASIK flap. These include slightly more inflammation after surgery, longer recovery time for vision to stabilize, and somewhat greater discomfort on the first night following the procedure. Lifting an Intralase flap for an enhancement is also somewhat more difficult than lifting a flap made with a standard microkeratome. These disadvantages are minor compared to the potential increased safety of using a laser rather than a blade to make the flap.

Although there are advantages to the IntraLase, the long-term safety record of a standard microkeratome and its continued success for many millions of patients may not justify a patient spending perhaps several hundred dollars more per eye for IntraLase. It is too early to tell if Femtosecond laser technology will become standard protocol or remain another option, but after having switched almost entirely to the IntraLase, I am quite happy with the results.

Phakic Intraocular Lenses

LASIK is usually highly successful in myopic patients up to approximately −10.00 D, and in hyperopic patients up to about +5.00 D. For those refractive errors outside of this range (−10.00 to +5.00), there may soon be another option. Although just recently approved in the United States, intraocular lenses have been used throughout the world for the correction of higher degrees of refractive errors. Intraocular lenses are similar to contact lenses, except that contact lenses are placed on the surface of the cornea, while intraocular lenses are placed inside the eye (intraocular). Because the intraocular lens (IOL) can be made in almost any power or prescription, it can conceivably correct almost every refractive error, even +10.00 to −20.00 and beyond. More importantly, the quality of vision would improve dramatically over that of contact lenses, spectacles, or even the excimer laser. Nevertheless, IOLs still have several problems that need to be resolved. The first problem is inherent in the procedure itself—surgery inside, rather than outside the eye. As in cataract and glaucoma surgery, the risk of infection is extremely small, but an infection inside the eye is far more serious than an infection on the surface of the eye, such as might occur in LASIK or Surface Ablation.

The second problem in IOL's to correct refractive errors is avoiding damage to the inside of the eye. Intraocular lenses have been used successfully for many years in cataract surgery to replace the cloudy lens, or cataract, that is removed. Following cataract removal, an IOL is placed in the space once occupied by the patient's own cloudy lens. If a patient does not have a cataract, an IOL (technically called a phakic IOL, after the Greek *phakos* or lens), the lens must be placed carefully inside the eye so that the delicate structures in the eye—the iris, lens, and cornea—are not traumatized or injured. A phakic IOL that corrects 15 diopters of myopia but rubs against the lens and causes a cataract or rubs against the surface of the cornea and causes clouding is not helping the patient.

In the next few years, more and more phakic IOLs that perform successfully should be available in the United States for eye surgeons and their patients. Two IOLs recently approved are the implantable contact lens, ICL, developed by Staar Surgical, and the Verisyse intraocular lens by American Medical Optics. These lenses have been extensively tested in the United States and have been used in patients throughout the world, providing excellent visual results contact lens (ICL), developed by Staar Surgical of Monrovia, California. This lens has been extensively tested in the United States and has been used in patients throughout the world, providing excellent visual results in highly myopic and hyperopic eyes with few complications.

Phakic IOLs should be a viable option in the near future. The more distant future will bring phakic IOLs that can be fine-tuned with a laser to correct under- and over-corrections overcorrections, ensuring 20/20 or better vision for almost all patients. Imagine a −15.00 D myope without glasses who cannot find the soap in the shower, then driving without glasses after twenty-minute phakic IOL surgery! This procedure will someday be a reality.

10

Presbyopia: New Solutions for Old Eyes

If you are under thirty-five, you can skip this chapter. If you are thirty-five to forty, I suggest you read it so you know what lies ahead as you approach optical old age. If you are forty or older, read it, understand it, and digest it. For patients age forty or older who are considering laser vision correction, modifying LVC to accommodate presbyopia may allow you to postpone reading glasses for many years.

Presbyopia, Greek for "old" *(presby)* and "sight" *(opia)* affects everyone as they age—that's 100% of all people. By age forty or fifty, but generally no later than fifty years of age, 100% of people will feel the need to adjust for reading. This adjustment may be as simple as holding print further away, using "longer arms," buying drugstore reading glasses, or, for the mild to moderately nearsighted, removing distance glasses to read.

For many patients, being over forty-five means wearing bifocals, with or without the telltale line, or having two pairs of glasses—one for distance and one for reading. For contact lens wearers, another option, other than reading glasses over the contacts, is one of the new bifocal or multifocal contact lenses. However, many contact lens wearers prefer monovision (also known as "blended vision"), where one eye is corrected for distance and the other for near, so that no reading glasses at all are needed. This system works especially well for people who work indoors, but can also work for people who drive or are out and about.

The same blended vision achieved in contact lenses can also be achieved with LVC. By correcting one eye for distance and the other for reading or computer, patients over age forty or forty-five may avoid reading glasses for many years. Understanding presbyopia and LVC options will help determine whether monovision is an option for you. Be sure to discuss this with your doctor.

Presbyopia occurs when hardening of the lens in your eye prevents it from changing shape to focus. In an ametropic person (one who does not need glasses for distance), the eye is naturally focused for distance, so no glasses are needed. For close vision, the ciliary muscles (the eye's focusing muscles), contract to thicken the jelly-like crystalline lens. The focusing process, called accommodation, gives the lens more power so that close objects, such as a book or a computer screen, become clear. The same process occurs when a camera focus is changed from a beautiful sunset in the distance to a friend or family member a few feet away. Presbyopia and accommodation are age dependent and affect both the myope and the presbyope, though the effect will be decidedly different depending on age. A fifty-year-old myope will usually be able to read, despite presbyopia, by removing his or her eyeglasses or contact lenses. By definition, a myope is focused at near, and a −3.00 D myope is focused at one-third of a meter (without correction), or about one foot—a convenient reading distance. Similarly, a −10.00 D myope is focused at one-tenth of a meter, or about four inches. Because holding reading material four inches away is not very convenient, and working at the computer four inches from the screen is impractical, a −10 D myope will need reading glasses or a bifocal to read at a normal distance. A −3.00 D myope will generally be comfortable reading or doing computer work without glasses.

To take this myopia discussion a step further, a −1.00 D myope will see clearly at one meter or three feet. A −1.00 D myope will have some clarity in reading a menu, price tag, or large letters without glasses. Reading glasses will be needed for regular reading, which is usually about sixteen inches from the face. The closer something is held, the stronger the focusing power or accommodation must be.

Hyperopes face presbyopia differently from myopes. Hyperopes become increasingly dependent on reading glasses as they age and do not have the myopes' luxury of being able to read by removing glasses. In fact, being over forty-five often uncovers a need for both reading and distance glasses. The reason for the hyperope's predicament is that, with age, the focusing or ciliary muscles lose their natural tone. In the young hyperope (under age forty), this tone, or focusing power, automatically self-corrects any distance problem by using more focusing power. Younger hyperopes often think they have perfect distance vision, but it is the result of continuous focusing by the ciliary muscles. With age, the focusing ability of the eye declines, and focusing for distance eventually exhausts the eyes' focusing power. This weakness in focusing, added to the increasing inelasticity of the eyes' natural lens (presbyopia), causes a need for correction in hyperopes for both distance and near. Bifocal spectacle or contact lenses correct both distance and near vision and are often the constant companion of the fifty-year-old hyperope.

As an example, consider John, age ten. His vision is 20/20 without glasses, and a refraction shows an eyeglass prescription of "plano"—an optical term indicating a zero, or no prescription. However, after John's eyes are dilated with eye drops, a repeat refraction shows a prescription of +3.00 D. The drops dilate the pupil and temporarily weaken the ciliary muscles, revealing "latent hyperopia" (hidden farsightedness) of the eye. Because the ciliary muscles of a ten-year-old have about ten diopters of focusing ability, John's ten diopters easily take care of the three diopters needed to see 20/20. Because he still has seven diopters remaining, he can read even the tiniest print at one-seventh of a meter or about five inches. Those ten diopters of focusing power decrease to about three diopters when John reaches age forty. A refraction with eye drops (a cycloplegic or "wet" refraction") will reveal that John is a +3.00 D hyperope. He must use all three diopters of focusing power to see distance and has nothing in reserve to focus up close. Eyeglasses or contact lenses of +3.00 D will give John perfect 20/20 for distance, and without his own formerly strong focusing reserve for seeing up close, John will need bifocals in order to read. Understanding the subtleties of presbyopia will help clarify what LVC can achieve for patients over forty, and what options are available to avoid reading glasses.

Options

1. If you are a myope over forty, you could have both eyes corrected for distance and use glasses for reading.

2. A myope over forty could have one eye, usually the dominant eye, corrected for distance and leave the second eye mildly myopic enough to read a price tag or menu without glasses. This "monovision" or "blended vision" system reduces, and often virtually eliminates, the need for reading glasses, making them necessary only for extensive reading or for reading extremely small print. For a mildly nearsighted forty-five-year-old, such as a –2.00 D myope, LVC might be needed for only one eye. The second, uncorrected eye would be perfect for reading without the use of glasses.

3. A hyperope over forty would generally be very satisfied if both eyes could be corrected for distance, requiring only reading glasses rather than full-time bifocals. For monovision (one eye for distance and one for near), the hyperope's eye designated for reading would need to be "overcorrected" and made nearsighted. If hyperopia is extreme, such as a refraction of +4.00 D or +5.00 D, excessive correction would be required to go from +5.00 D to –1.00 D or –2.00 D and quality of vision might suffer. So, depending on how farsighted you are, you may have to settle for distance vision without the option of monovision.

If you and your ophthalmologist decide that monovision is an option, remember that there are disadvantages. Monovision reduces depth perception, often barely perceptible to most patients, but sometimes annoying to others. It may, therefore, be most appropriate for patients who work in an office rather than for those who do much driving or play sports. For these activities, part-time eyeglasses may be necessary for distance. Because of these drawbacks, monovision may not be suitable for some professionals, such as athletes, pilots, and truck drivers. In addition, some people simply are unable to adjust to monovision.

Monovision can be experienced before committing to it in LVC. Your eye doctor can adequately mimic the effect of monovision by placing contact lenses, each with a different power, in each eye—one for far (usually your dominant eye) and one for near. You need not be a contact lens wearer to experience monovision. Your eye doctor can insert the lenses in the morning, allowing you to go to work or do errands, and remove them later in the day. Even a brief wearing should give you some idea if you would be comfortable with monovision.

Monovision can delay full-time reading glasses well into your fifties and sixties, but eventually, reading glasses will become necessary. Until then, monovision is an effective solution for many patients, especially those whose professions demand a great deal of reading, such as lawyers and accountants. Discuss monovision with your eye doctor and try to experience it with contact lenses if you are unsure.

11

Conductive Keratoplasty (CK): New Hope for Some Hyperopes and Presbyopes

Approved by the FDA in early 2002, conductive keratoplasty (CK) is a nonlaser, minimally invasive procedure for low-to-moderate hyperopes over forty. CK is also used to treat patients who otherwise have normal distance vision, but because of their presbyopia, must wear reading glasses. CK has also been used to fine-tune hyperopia or astigmatism resulting from previous LVC or cataract surgery. Instead of a laser, CK uses spots of radio-frequency energy, placed in one, two, or three circles of eight spots each, with the spot pattern around the circumference of the cornea (see Figure 9). The energy is delivered to the cornea by a tiny probe inserted into the stroma—the middle layer of the cornea. Each burst of energy takes about a half-second and is rendered painless by anesthetic eye drops. After the spots of radio-frequency energy are applied, the center of the cornea steepens, correcting the hyperopia, or farsightedness. Treatment is applied in eight evenly spaced spots in a ring around the circumference of the cornea. The more rings of spots there are, the more the hyperopia is corrected. To correct a refractive error of +0.75 D to +1.00 D, a circle of eight spots is applied. Correcting +1.00 D to +2.00 D requires sixteen spots, while +2.00 D to +3.00 D requires twenty-four spots (a newly improved technique for performing CK may make only eight spots enough for most patients). The FDA recently approved CK for the correction of presbyopia in patients who only need reading glasses, making it the only surgical procedure approved by the FDA for this purpose (patients who wear bifocals may do better with LVC). Although CK can correct hyperopia, the correction of presbyopia—a more widespread condition, will likely be the primary use of CK.

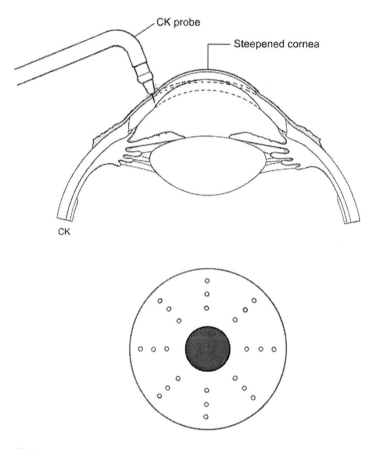

Fig. 9

Fig 9. Conductive Keratoplasty (CK) steepens the cornea with the use of spots of radio frequency energy.

A CK treatment for presbyopia is performed on the nondominant eye only, steepening the shape of the cornea to make the eye near-sighted. In most cases, one or two rings of eight spots each will create enough nearsightedness for reading price tags, menus, cell phones, wristwatches, computer screens, and newspapers. For reading exten-sively, or for reading very small type or in poor lighting, many patients will still require part-time reading glasses.

CK has many advantages and some disadvantages. The main advan-tage is safety. Although the CK probe penetrates the cornea, akin to acupuncture, there is no cutting, no blade, no flap, and no laser. The radio-frequency energy creates a minuscule and localized area of heat that shrinks the collagen tissue of the cornea, in effect tightening the outside of the cornea and steepening the center. Of the three hundred and fifty-five eyes treated with CK in the FDA study, none had com-plications or adverse events.

Another advantage for CK is that it can be done in your eye doctor's office rather than in a laser center or laser room. Some patients may find this environment more convenient and comfortable, preferring the familiar surroundings of their ophthalmologist's office to a high-tech laser center. Most CK patients do not need someone to accom-pany them home. Care after CK is minimal, often consisting of only a few drops of antibiotic or artificial tear drops.

CK can also be used after other eye procedures, such as LASIK and cataract surgery, when some residual astigmatism or hyperopia may still be still present. With astigmatism, one or two CK spots is all that may be needed to reshape the cornea to a more rounded and less oval (astigmatic) shape, thereby improving uncorrected vision with a sim-ple, minimally invasive procedure.

However, CK has two main disadvantages. The procedure may cre-ate astigmatism, which may counteract the improvement in hyperopia or presbyopia. Astigmatism occurs if the spot pattern is not precisely centered around the circumference of the pupil, or if the spots are not all at the same depth, do not have the same energy, or do not heal the same way. The spot pattern is transferred to the cornea with the help of a blue dye and marker. Because this pattern is centered "freehand" on the cornea by the ophthalmologist, it is almost impossible for it to be exactly centered every time. Fortunately, small centering discrepancies cause only negligible amounts of astigmatism. If larger amounts develop, a follow-up CK procedure that places one or two balancing spots at the appropriate position on your cornea to cancel out the astigmatism will usually correct the problem.

Another disadvantage of CK is that the effect of the procedure tends to wane over several years as the aging process continues, so touch-ups may be necessary every three to five years. This fading is not as bad as in botox treatments, which last only a few months, or teeth whitening, which fades away in about a year or so. Most ophthalmologists will charge a reduced fee for CK touch-up procedures. CK is best described as an antiaging procedure that reverses aging but does not stop it. CK can restore vision to the level that existed prior to wearing glasses in presbyopic and hyperopic patients. If you want to turn back the clock and eliminate dependence on reading glasses, CK may be your answer.

Several other technologies currently under study may provide a surgical solution to presbyopia. As of right now, however, CK and monovision may be the best solutions for many patients over forty-five who want to minimize their dependence on distance and/or reading glasses. A permanent surgical solution to presbyopia remains for the future, but studies using the excimer laser to create a multifocal cornea in LASIK show promise. Intraocular multifocal lenses are being tested in clinical trials for the presbyope without cataracts, so more help is on the way.

12

Conclusion

According to the old saying, the eyes are the windows to the soul—you can look into someone's eyes and know what they may be thinking or feeling or whether you should trust them.

As debatable as that saying may be, there is little debate that the eyes are also the windows to your own world. They look. They provide you with the world, and everything you see in it. LASIK, PRK, or LASEK can improve that world and free you from total dependence on eyeglasses or contact lenses. Today's diagnostic and surgical advances have created an environment of safe and effective laser vision correction.

Before considering LVC, remember the mantra—realistic expectations. Having realistic expectations is the key to being satisfied following LVC. Because not everyone achieves 20/20 or even 20/40 vision, LVC may not eliminate glasses from your life completely. Realistic expectations means anyone considering "no more glasses" must accept the likelihood that glasses may be necessary for some tasks—to drive at night or see *Les Miserables* from the back of the theater. After reading this book, you should have a clear idea whether laser vision correction is right for you. It is easy to understand the many benefits of LVC, but you must also understand the potential complications. You must select a surgeon with whom you are comfortable, have a thorough eye examination, and discuss your options. You must also be willing to assume some risk. Even as safe as it is, LVC is still surgery and always carries risk. With modern advances in instruments and the femtosecond laser to create the flap, and in excimer lasers to reshape the cornea, LASIK is safer than it has ever been. For those patients who want to eliminate flap risks, Surface Ablation is a good option. By knowing the pros and cons of LVC and having realistic expectations, most patients will experience results that far exceed their expectations.

APPENDIX A

What to Ask Your Surgeon

However you find your surgeon—through word of mouth, the Yellow Pages, radio, television, or newspaper advertisement, referral to an eye surgeon by your regular optometrist, or staying with your regular ophthalmologist—there are certain credentials to look for and questions to ask:

1. Always look for a board-certified physician. Board certification is the medical profession's accepted form of accreditation. This information is usually found on one of your doctor's diplomas or can be obtained from the American Academy of Ophthalmology or the American Board of Ophthalmology.

2. Ask for additional certification of competence in laser vision surgery. Many ophthalmologists today started practice before the excimer laser was developed and approved by the FDA in 1995. Training programs and fellowships are conducted by the American Academy of Ophthalmology, the American Society of Cataract and Refractive Surgeons, and other organizations, as well as by a hospital's department of ophthalmology. The manufacturers of lasers and microkeratomes also provide laser vision surgery training certification. Simply asking your ophthalmologist about his or her specific training in LASIK, epi-LASIK, PRK, or LASEK is the best way to begin finding out the extent of an individual surgeon's credentials.

3. Check with your state medical board to see if the surgeon has had multiple malpractice suits. Keep in mind that in today's litigious society, even the best physicians may have been sued for malpractice. The red flag occurs when there have been multiple lawsuits per year. If they have more than one lawsuit per year, you should ask for an explanation.

4. Experience is one of the most important issues. Studies indicate that LASIK, epi-LASIK, PRK, and LASEK each have learning curves, and those doctors who have performed more than one hundred procedures generally have a lower complication rate than surgeons who have performed less than one hundred. This is at best, a very general rule, because an experienced surgeon, well trained in cataract or glaucoma surgery, may have a much shorter learning curve in learning LVC than a novice surgeon who is experienced only in LVC procedures.

5. Ask your surgeon whether he or she tracks outcomes. What percentage of patients achieves 20/20 or 20/40, and what percentage has any loss of best corrected visual acuity (BCVA)? Ask about their success and complication rates. Obviously, you want a surgeon with a high success rate and a low complication rate. Although every laser vision correction surgeon has had patients with complications, it's important to know the frequency of complications, how the complications were resolved, and whether the final visual outcomes were good. Ask about enhancement rates—the average is less than 5%. Ask about your suitability for LVC. By reading this book, you should better understand the results of the tests done by your doctor to determine your suitability for LVC. Review your refraction, corneal thickness, curvature and topography, and the general health of your eyes. Review any medical problems that may affect your suitability. Be an educated consumer, as suggested by Marcy Syms.

While the above guidelines are important, nothing is foolproof. Personal chemistry is important. Don't dismiss your intuition or gut feelings. Do you trust this physician? Don't be reluctant to ask questions about experience and certification. Ask as many questions as it takes for you to decide if LVC and your eye doctor are right for you. Your eye doctor should emphasize realistic expectations and discuss potential problems and complications. To trust your vision correction surgeon, you must have confidence in your own feelings. You are looking for a good surgeon, not a good salesperson.

Extend your trust barometer to your ophthalmologist's staff. The staff should be experienced, well-trained, and as compassionate and considerate as is your doctor. In many offices and laser centers, you will be dealing with a host of people—the person performing the surgery may not be the one doing most of the testing and most of the follow up care.

In that case, make sure the following questions are adequately addressed:

- Who will be your main contact at the office or center?

- Will the surgeon evaluate your eye exam results and speak with you before surgery?

- Who will perform your the follow-up exams? With rare exceptions, your surgeon should see you on your first postoperative visit.

- What are the qualifications of the person performing the pre-and postoperative exams?

- How many follow-up visits will be needed?

- What restrictions will you have?

APPENDIX B

FDA Approval

The Food and Drug Administration does not approve medical procedures; it approves medical devices. It is responsible for assessing and affirming the safety and efficacy of products used by health care providers. The FDA approves a drug or device for a specific use. Devices and drugs, when approved by the FDA for the treatment of a specific condition or disorder, can only be sold in the United States for that purpose. This approved use is called an indication.

Five different excimer lasers approved by the FDA since 1995 are currently in use in the United States. The indications are for either PRK or LASIK, although some have been approved for both, and the indications also include refraction ranges. In general, approval has been given to correct hyperopia up to +6.00 D, myopia up to −14.00 D, and for varying degrees of astigmatism. Specific prescription ranges are approved for each brand of excimer laser. If a doctor uses a laser for a prescription outside of the approved indications or uses a laser for LASIK that is only approved for PRK, he or she is engaged in an "off-label" use. The FDA does not regulate or police the practice or the practitioners of medicine. A physician is allowed to use an approved device for an "off-label" procedure, as long as the device, including hardware and software, has not been modified from what was originally FDA approved. "Off-label" is not a reason for suspicion. Many medical breakthroughs have been attained by physicians using a drug or device for something other than the approved use. In most cases, it means that insufficient data has been accumulated for the indication to be approved by the FDA. For some lasers used for LASIK, the FDA initially gave premarket approval (PMA) only for use in PRK—use in LASIK was "off-label." Eventually, full FDA approval was granted for LASIK. Almost all lasers now have been approved for LASIK. As of this writing, epi-LASIK and LASEK are off-label. After deliberation, the FDA decided that because different instruments and solutions are used and different laser parameters are employed, LASEK would require separate approval. This should be forthcoming from the FDA in the near future, after clinical studies are completed.

The microkeratome received approval in the 1980s for automated lamellar keratoplasty (ALK), a precursor to modern LASIK. Because the modern-day microkeratome functions in much the same way in LASIK as it did in ALK, no additional approval was required.

Often, the FDA approves a laser up to a certain diopter range and sets a software "flag" above that range to let the surgeon know that the indication is off-label—not within the approved range. Sometimes the FDA, feeling it has evidence about safety and effectiveness, requires a "hard lock," in which case the ablation cannot be performed above a specific range without changing the software. In these cases, the surgeon may decide to "double card" the patient. This means, for example, if the surgeon wants to obtain a −12.00 D correction, he or she may perform a −10.00 D ablation and a −2.00 D ablation. Double-card is an off-label use and must be specified as such. Double card procedures are uncommon today because of a wider range of refractions corrected with one card and other options, such as intraocular lenses, for very high prescriptions.

APPENDIX C

A Century of Study—A Short History of Refractive Surgery

The excimer laser, approved for use in vision surgery by the Food and Drug Administration in 1995, heralded a new era in eye care. Soon, people would be able to throw away their eyeglasses and contact lenses. The future was here. Most people did not know that refractive surgery and other means of eliminating glasses were not new, with roots going back more than half a century when the foundation was laid for the safe and effective "breakthrough" that now cures hundreds of thousands of patients each year.

In 1869, Hermann Snellen—the same ophthalmologist who devised the Snellen chart and applied the term 20/20 to visual acuity measurement—published a paper proposing that making incisions on the cornea would change its shape and correct severe astigmatism. By the late 1890s, attempts to correct such astigmatism through corneal incisions were described in separate studies by W. H. Bates in the United States and L. J. Lans in Germany. Bates's early contribution to the evolution of vision surgery is notable now because it seems so out-of-character with his later career: he eventually proposed that all refractive errors derived from eye strain and an "abnormal condition of the mind," for which he prescribed physical and mental exercises. Bates proposed his theories in a 1920 book, that even though long rejected by most eye doctors, is still reprinted—a testimony to the search for an alternative to eyeglasses and contact lenses. Lans performed several variations of corneal surgery, all designed to alter astigmatism, on rabbits. The principles of his century-old research formed the basis of modern-day radial keratotomy (from *kera*, meaning cornea and *otomy*, to cut). Lans discovered that radial incisions in the anterior (outside) surface of the cornea flattened the cornea.

Snellen, Bates, and Lans were initially drawn to refractive eye surgery as a means to correct visual impairment from keratoconus, a condition in which the cornea becomes extremely steep and irregular, almost cone-shaped with vision poorly corrected by eyeglasses. During the 1930s, Japanese ophthalmologist Tutomo Sato noticed something unique in the progression of keratoconus. In some patients, the cornea stretched to such an extent that minute cracks or tears developed in the back of the cornea, allowing fluid from inside the eye to seep into the cornea, causing it to swell and blister. The result was pain, profuse watering, and light sensitivity lasting several days. These symptoms dissipated spontaneously when the cracks in the cornea healed. Sato found that, in some patients, the thin scar that formed in the area of the tear caused the cone-shaped cornea to flatten, decreasing myopia and astigmatism and improving vision. Sato tried to mimic what happened naturally in some patients by making cuts in the back of the cornea in an attempt to flatten it. The technique required making dozens of radial—radiating from the center like spokes in a wheel—cuts inside or in the posterior part of the cornea. Sato continued to perform this very exacting surgery until the 1950s when contact lenses became available in Japan. While Sato's technique demonstrated that flattening the cornea corrected vision, the surgery was tragically flawed. He, and other ophthalmologists of that era, failed to recognize the importance of the endothelium (the layer of cells on the inside of the cornea), which prevents fluids in the eye from entering the cornea. Ten to twenty years after their surgery, many of his patients suffered serious loss of sight from corneal swelling, resulting from the severe damage unwittingly inflicted on the endothelium.

Ophthalmologists have since learned to respect the endothelial cells that line the back of the cornea when performing refractive and other types of ophthalmic surgery, such as for cataracts and glaucoma. In the post-Sato era of vision correction surgery, ophthalmologists realized they could make incisions only on the surface of the cornea, not on the inside. This epiphany did not occur until the 1970s, when Svyatislov Fyodorov, an ophthalmologist in the USSR, modified Sato's technique.

As the story reads, a patient of Fyodorov's, a nearsighted teenage boy, had his glasses broken during a fight and several shards of the glass lenses pierced his cornea. Fyodorov discovered that after the cuts in the cornea healed, the cornea flattened and the patient gained normal vision. His myopia gradually faded away. The Soviet ophthalmologist was familiar with Sato's work and began experiments on rabbits. Five years later, he performed radial keratotomies on humans. By the end of the decade, Fyodorov had fully developed the RK procedure—a series of radial incisions in the cornea that flattened it and corrected modest amounts of myopia. In 1978, American ophthalmologist Leo Borres performed the first RK procedure in the United States.

RK Becomes Popular

By the end of the 1980s, several studies showed the efficacy of RK for myopia. More than one hundred thousand patients received the treatment. The complex surgery required eight to sixteen incisions on the surface of the cornea. The surgery corrected modest amounts of myopia, but lacked the predictability of LASIK and had a longer healing time.

As the dawn of the laser era grew closer, it became obvious that a concentrated beam of light was a more precise surgical tool than a handheld scalpel for corneal microsurgery. The laser procedure still had a long road to travel before the profession became convinced it was practical and not just science fiction.

Technology Convergence

In fact, the road to LASIK began decades before the invention of the laser. In 1949, Colombian ophthalmologist José Barraquer developed lamellar (layered) corneal surgery, in which the cornea's shape was changed by removing a contact lens-shaped disk from the front portion of the cornea. The instrument invented by Barraquer, the micro-keratome, was based on a carpenter's plane. Using the microkeratome, Barraquer removed a disk from the front portion of the cornea, froze it, and reshaped it on a mechanical lathe called a cryolathe. The newly shaped disk was then placed back on the cornea, thus correcting the refractive error—similar to how LASIK corrects refractive errors. Bar-raquer spent thirteen years experimenting and fine-tuning his new operation, lamellar keratoplasty. While he, too, originally developed the surgery as a cure for keratoconus, he expanded the indications to include myopia and hyperopia in healthy eyes. By the mid-80s, the cryolathe had become automated. In 1985, Casimir Swinger, a New York ophthalmologist, developed nonfreeze keratomileusis, a method using the microkeratome to change the cornea's shape without freez-ing. In 1987, Luis Ruiz, a protégé of Barraquer, developed an auto-mated microkeratome that led to automated lamellar keratoplatsy (ALK), which corrected high degrees of myopia and hyperopia. Before the automated microkeratome, the procedure lacked predictable out-comes because not all surgeons could master the skills necessary for the complicated manual microkeratome. ALK offered more stable results than RK for patients with high myopia and hyperopia, and, though it has been abandoned in the wake of LASIK, it paved the way for mod-ern laser vision correction. The real breakthrough in laser vision correc-tion came in 1983 when Dr. Stephen L. Trokel, a Columbia University ophthalmologist who was working with IBM physicist Dr. S. R. Srinivasan, proposed the revolutionary idea that the excimer laser that IBM used to etch circuitry in computer microchips could reshape the cornea. To demonstrate the precision and accuracy of the excimer laser, Srinivasan took a remarkable and much reprinted photograph demonstrating how the excimer laser could cut precise notches in a human hair. Dr. Trokel then teamed up with California physicist Charles R. Munnerlyn, and the two painstakingly developed algorithms and computer models that indicated how much tissue should be removed to correct different degrees of nearsightedness. Other ophthalmologists, such as Louisiana's Dr. Marguerite B. McDonald, a renowned corneal surgeon and researcher, conducted independent studies that proved Trokel's theory—the excimer laser could safely vaporize corneal tissue without damaging any surrounding tissue, permitting a predictable change in corneal curvature and the refraction of the eye.

In 1987, Theodore W. Seiler, a German ophthalmologist, performed the world's first PRK on a normally sighted human eye, and the next year Dr. McDonald performed the first PRK in the United States. Years of carefully documented and controlled clinical trials followed until 1995, when the FDA approved Summit Technology's excimer laser for PRK to correct nearsightedness. The following year the FDA granted approval to VISX Corporation's excimer laser, also for PRK. Since then, hundreds of thousands of PRK procedures have been successfully performed worldwide.

LASIK was born in 1989 when Italian ophthalmologist Lucio Buratto used the excimer laser to ablate tissue on the underside of a cornea disk made during ALK. This was the moment when ALK met PRK. Modern LASIK quickly evolved, and in 1991 Stephen Brint, an ophthalmologist with Summit Technology, performed the first LASIK as it is practiced today.

Since 1991 ophthalmologists and scientists have improved the workings of the laser, the microkeratomes, and introduced new tools, such as the femtosecond laser and the aberrometer for custom laser treatments. The result has been safer, more accurate, and highly predictable vision correction surgery. "No more glasses" became a reality.

Glossary

A

Ablate: To remove by vaporizing tissue. In laser vision correction, it describes the action of the excimer laser beam in reshaping the cornea by removing corneal tissue.

Accommodation: The process by which the eye increases its focusing power to see close objects, such as the type on this page. Accommodation takes place through the contraction of the ciliary muscles, which control the shape of the crystalline lens, becoming thicker to focus up close, and thinner to focus for objects far away.

Aqueous Humor: The transparent, water-like liquid filling the space between the cornea and the crystalline lens. It nourishes the cornea, iris, and lens and helps maintain intraocular pressure and the shape of the cornea.

Astigmatic Keratotomy (AK): Vision surgery for correcting astigmatism. Similar to RK (radial keratotomy) for myopia, it is often performed at the same time as cataract surgery to correct astigmatism. With the advent of laser vision surgery, AK alone is rarely performed today.

Astigmatism: Common refractive error, in which the cornea is oval or football-shaped, as opposed to being spherical like a baseball.

Automated Lamellar Keratoplasty (ALK): Vision correcting surgery using a gear-driven microkeratome to create a corneal flap, and then using the keratome to remove stromal corneal tissue to reshape it and correct a refractive error. The procedure is rarely performed today, but the principles are the same ones used for LASIK

B

Bandage Soft Contact Lens: A soft contact lens with little or no prescription, used like a bandage for comfort, and to promote healing of the corneal surface after PRK or LASEK.

BCVA (Best Corrected Visual Acuity): Maximum visual acuity, obtained through the use of optical devices, such as eyeglasses or contact lenses. BCVA is an important benchmark for eyesight and the health of the eye.

Bowman's Membrane: A microthin layer of tissue beneath the epithelium of the cornea. Bowman's layer separates the epithelium from the stroma. Microstria involve microscopic folds or cracks in Bowman's membrane.

C

Ciliary Muscles: Muscular tissue surrounding the iris that controls the expansion and contraction of the crystalline lens, enabling it to focus.

Concave Lens: A lens that is thinner in the center and thicker at the edge, used to correct myopia. Opposite of convex.

Convex Lens: A lens that is thicker in the center and thinner at the edge, used to correct hyperopia. Opposite of concave.

Cornea: The clear, front part of the eye. The cornea bends or refracts light that enters the eye. Laser vision surgery reshapes the cornea to correct refractive errors.

Crystalline Lens: The lens of the eye, located behind the iris; has the ability to change shape to provide the eye with most of its focusing power. A lens, cloudy from age, is called a cataract.

D

Descemet's Membrane: Next to last layer of the cornea. Supports the endothelium and acts as a barrier so that aqueous fluid does not get into the cornea, and cause swelling and loss of clarity. It is rarely affected by laser vision surgery.

Diffuse Lamellar Keratitis (DLK): A temporary inflammatory reaction beneath the LASIK corneal flap. Condition resembles swirling, shifting sand. DLK is also called "Sands of the Sahara." Prompt treatment with corticosteroid eyedrops should prevent adverse effects.

Diopter (D): The measurement determining degrees of refractive error, similar to measuring length in feet and weight in pounds. A negative (–) diopter value signifies myopia, and a positive (+) diopter value signifies hyperopia.

Dry Eye Syndrome: A common condition that occurs when the eyes do not produce enough tears to keep the eyes moist and comfortable. Symptoms can include stinging, burning, foreign-body sensation, and intermittent blurring of vision. Severe dry eye can preclude patients from having laser vision surgery. In some patients, it can be a temporary postoperative condition after LASIK.

E

Endothelium: The fifth layer of the cornea. Consists of a layer of cells that line the inside of the cornea. The endothelium acts as a semipermeable barrier, keeping the cornea correctly hydrated. Not invaded during laser vision surgery.

Epithelium: The first, outer layer of cells of the cornea; the eye's first defense against infection. The epithelium is always invaded during laser vision surgery, but completely regenerates within about a week following PRK.

Excimer laser: A cool ultraviolet laser used in refractive surgery to ablate corneal tissue. Vaporizes specific areas of corneal tissue without damaging surrounding tissue.

F

Farsightedness: Hyperopia.

Focus: What the eye does when it accommodates. The ability of the cornea to refract light, and the crystalline lens to expand or contract to aim that light onto the retina.

H

Haze: Commonly known as corneal haze, postoperative clouding of the cornea that occasionally follows laser vision surgery, especially PRK for higher prescriptions. Often temporary. Treated with prolonged use of steroid eye drops and rarely causes serious vision problems.

Hyperopia (farsighted): Refractive error in which light rays are focused behind the retina due to a relatively short eye or a flat cornea. In younger patients with ciliary muscle reserve, self-corrects without glasses with contraction of these muscles.

I

Informed Consent Form: A document disclosing the risks, benefits, and alternatives to a procedure. Patients are required to read, understand, and sign an informed consent form prior to laser vision surgery.

Iris: The colored ring of tissue surrounding the pupil and suspended behind the cornea in front of the lens. Muscles in the iris control pupil size.

K

Keratectomy: The surgical removal of corneal tissue.

Keratotomy: A surgical incision in the cornea.

Keratitis: Inflammation of the cornea. Diffuse lamellar keratitis (DLK) is one example.

Kerato: Pertaining to the cornea. Latin for cornea.

Keratoconus: A hereditary degenerative corneal disease characterized by an irregular thinning of the cornea, leading to a cone-shaped protrusion of the cornea. Keratoconus generally occurs in patients in their thirties, resulting in blurred and distorted vision that, in severe cases, may require rigid contact lenses to restore vision. LASIK is not recommended at this time for patients with keratoconus.

Keratomileusis: Sculpting the cornea. From the Greek *keratos* (cornea) and *mileusis* (carving).

L

Laser: Acronym for light amplification by stimulated emission of radiation. As a surgical instrument, the laser produces a powerful beam of light that vaporizes tissue.

LASEK: Acronym for laser epithelial keratomileusis, a newer technique for vision surgery. Instead of making a corneal flap with the microkeratome, the surgeon uses a diluted alcohol solution or other means to loosen and retain the epithelium, which is then used to cover the cornea after the ablation. LASEK combines principles of both LASIK and PRK.

LASIK: Acronym for laser-assisted in situ keratomileusis. A surgical procedure in which a corneal, stromal flap is created with a microkeratome, followed by excimer laser ablation to reshape the corneal stroma.

Lens: The normally clear structure behind the iris and pupil that helps focus light onto the retina. Also called the crystalline lens. In optics, any piece of transparent material with the ability to bend light rays predictably, such as spectacle lenses or contact lenses.

M

Micron (μ): Unit of measure equal to one thousandth of a millimeter. Used to measure the amount of tissue ablated during laser vision correction. Removal of 12 microns of tissue generally corrects one diopter of myopia.

Microkeratome: A surgical instrument used to create a corneal flap during LASIK.

Monovision: A modification of vision correction during which one eye is corrected for near vision and the other for distance vision. Often used as a solution for presbyopia. Can be achieved through contact lenses, vision surgery, or eyeglasses.

Myopia (nearsightedness): Refractive error with clear near vision and blurry distance vision. Caused by a cornea that is too steep or an eye that is too long. Laser vision surgery corrects myopia by flattening the cornea.

N

Nearsightedness: Myopia.

Nomogram: An adjustment made to the data entered into the excimer laser to give the best results for each patient. To minimize the chances of an overcorrection in a myopic patient, a nomogram will normally deduct a small amount of laser correction for older patients and those with high prescriptions and add a small amount for hyperopic patients to minimize undercorrections.

O

Ophthalmologist: A physician specializing in the diagnosis and medical and surgical treatment of vision disorders and eye disease.

Optician: Eye care provider skilled in making and fitting eyeglasses. In some states, may also fit contact lenses.

Optometrist: Eye care professional and doctor of optometry who can diagnose and treat many eye diseases and disorders of the visual system. Unlike ophthalmologists, optometrists are not physicians and are not trained or licensed to perform surgery.

Overcorrection: In vision correction surgery, when the achieved amount of correction is more than desired.

P

PRK: Acronym for photorefractive keratectomy, a surface ablation procedure that removes the surface epithelium before the stroma is ablated and reshaped by a computer-controlled excimer laser.

Presbyopia (Old eyes): The ability to focus on near objects is diminished when the crystalline lens loses elasticity. Presbyopia is a natural symptom of aging, occurring in nearly 100% of the population between the ages of forty-five and fifty.

Pupil: Opening in the center of the iris that regulates the amount of light entering the eye. The pupil enlarges, or dilates, in dim light and gets smaller, or constricts, in bright light.

R

Radial Keratotomy (RK): Surgical procedure designed to correct myopia by flattening the cornea using radial incisions. Rarely performed today with the advent of laser vision surgery.

Refraction: Tests to determine the refractive power of the eye. Also refers to the bending of light as it passes through a lens. Used to determine a prescription for eyeglasses.

Refractive Errors: Results when light is not focused precisely to a point on the retina. Hyperopia occurs when a point of light lands behind the retina, myopia occurs when light lands in front, and astigmatism occurs when light forms a diffuse focal point near the retina.

Refractive Power: Degree of the power of an object, such as the cornea or lens, to bend light as light passes through it.

Retina: Membrane lining the inner wall of the eye that converts light entering the eye into electrical impulses that are sent to the brain and converted into images.

S

Sclera: The white of the eye—white, fibrous, protective outer layer of the eye.

Snellen Visual Acuity Chart: Used to measure vision, from which the term 20/20 vision is derived.

Striae: Folds or wrinkles in the corneal flap; complication of LASIK that can be corrected several ways, including lifting, stretching, and repositioning the flap.

Stroma: Middle and thickest layer of the cornea. In vision correction surgery, the stroma is reshaped, or sculpted, to correct refractive errors.

Surface Ablation: General term for an excimer laser treatment performed on the surface of the cornea as opposed to LASIK, where the treatment is under a corneal flap.

T

Trephine: Round cookie cutter-like instrument used in LASEK to hold a diluted alcohol solution to loosen the surface epithelium.

U

Undercorrection: In vision correction surgery, when the achieved amount of correction is less than desired.

V

Visual Acuity: Patient's level of vision, usually based on the Snellen eye chart.

W

Wavefront Technology: Diagnostic scanning systems using waves of infrared light to give a more complete picture of the aberrations and imperfections of the eye, including the refractive error.

Z

Zonules: Fibers attaching the crystalline lens to the ciliary body muscles.

Index

978-0-595-35421-4
0-595-35421-1